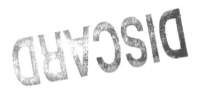

The Art of
Taking It Easy

HOW TO COPE WITH
BEARS, TRAFFIC, AND THE REST
OF LIFE'S STRESSORS

The Art
of Taking
It Easy

Dr. Brian King

PSYCHOLOGIST AND COMEDIAN

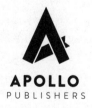

APOLLO
PUBLISHERS

The Art of Taking It Easy:

How to Cope with Bears, Traffic, and the Rest of Life's Stressors

Copyright © 2019 by Dr. Brian King

Apollo Publishers books may be purchased for educational, business, or sales promotional use. Special editions may be made available upon request. For details, contact Apollo Publishers at info@apollopublishers.com.

Visit our website at www.apollopublishers.com.

Library of Congress Cataloging-in-Publication Data is available on file.

Print ISBN: 978-1-948062-46-6

Ebook ISBN: 978-1-948062-47-3

Printed in the United States of America.

For Alyssa,

———————————

Although it is impossible for me to protect you from all the bad things that happen in life, I can definitely teach you the skills to cope with whatever comes your way.

Contents

Are You Happy?

hope so, I really do. And I'm not just saying that to get you on my side either; the happiness of other people has always been very important to me.

Comedians frequently open a joke by saying, "And now, a little about me," so let me start by telling you a little about myself. As the book cover says, I am Dr. Brian King, although I really only use my title as a stage name. I am a pretty casual guy so I usually just go by Brian. Besides, I've never been comfortable calling myself "Dr. King"—that name has already been taken.[1]

As a public speaker with a doctorate in psychology, I have been traveling the country teaching audiences about happiness, the benefits of humor, and how to manage stress for nearly a decade. These subjects are very interrelated, as managing stress is key to happiness, and humor contributes to them both. I've devoted a good chunk of my life to teaching people how to overcome stress and live happier lives. I also perform stand-up comedy, an art form with the sole purpose of making people happy. Comedians screw

---

1 If you don't get this reference, perhaps you were skipping school in February?

this up all the time, but at least that is the intent.

I seem to have an ability to present research-based information in a humorous context, and this has been the key to my success as a speaker, and now, an author. In 2016 I published a book, *The Laughing Cure*, all about the physical and emotional benefits of humor and laughter, which has been met with positive reviews and, I am told, has helped at least a few people become happier.

When I look back on my life, of course I see things that I could have done differently, but I was always concerned about the happiness of others. In high school I was part of a peer counseling program, based on the idea that a troubled student would prefer talking to another student rather than an adult in a position of authority.[2] In college, I volunteered with an organization that helped organize and train a new generation of those student mentors. I also volunteered my time to a few charities, and worked in a home for emotionally disturbed children. When I became a public speaker, I took the opportunity to pursue something I had been interested in all my life.

So yes, I am interested in your happiness.

I realize that in choosing to pick up this book, there is a chance that happiness is something you may be struggling with. Maybe you are coping with some terrible circumstances or wrestling with anxiety and depression. After all, these are our most

---

2 Peer Assistance and Leadership is a great idea, and an awesome experience. See http://palusa.org for more information.

common mental disorders.[3] Perhaps you are looking for answers, hoping that somehow these pages may contain that magical key to overcoming whatever you are dealing with. If this is the case, I don't want to discourage you from reading further, but I don't think any book has all the answers. (Unless you are looking up a phone number, in which case I know a great book for that. And what is it, 1997 where you live?)

Certainly reading a book is no substitute for professional help, but you may find some value in what I have to share.

Let me be clear, nobody is happy all the time. In fact, to be happy all the time is indicative of a disorder.[4] Healthy people fluctuate in their emotions. We have highs, we have lows, and overall, we have a general level of affect that would describe our usual emotional state. If we averaged all of our ups and downs, we'd have an emotional equilibrium, if you will.[5] Like any human trait, we would expect this to vary from person to person, and it does. Some of us are naturally quite happy, experiencing an overall high level of affect, some of us unfortunately experience much more down time, but most of us are somewhere in the middle: a level of happiness that my dad would describe as "Can't complain."

When I introduce myself to seminar audiences, I often start by stating that I am quite happy, and this is true. I am definitely not the happiest person I have ever met, but I am above average in this

---

3 Anxiety disorders are the most common mental illness in the United States, affecting forty million adults age eighteen and older, 18 percent of the population. (Source: National Institute of Mental Health, http://www.nimh.nih.gov/health/statistics/prevalence/any-anxiety-disorder-among-adults.shtml.)

4 Angelman syndrome.

5 For a great summary on modern happiness research and theory, see Sonja Lyubomirsky, *The How of Happiness: A Scientific Approach to Getting the Life You Want* (New York, NY: Penguin, 2008).

regard. I know how to take it easy. For the cover of my last book, my brother, Jon, provided the following endorsement: "Brian has been unaffected by stress since I met him when he was five. I think he tapped into how to manage stress and live on his own terms at an early age." Generally speaking, I live a pretty stress-free life, and as a result I experience more emotional highs than lows. This does not mean that I have not dealt with my share of adverse events; I absolutely have. Bad things happen all the time, but what ultimately makes the difference in our lives is how we deal with those situations.

With the growing field of Positive Psychology, there has been a lot of research on what makes people happy and how some are able to handle stress better than others. Certain characteristics and behaviors have been identified and somehow, I managed to grow to adulthood with a good set of skills for achieving happiness. In other words, I practice what I preach. For this reason, I tend to use personal examples whenever I can (and sometimes I just straight make them up; after all, I am a comedian). The doctorate in psychology helps too, but I'll let you in on a not-so-secret secret: Not all psychologists are positive. A lot of psychologists suffer from depression too.

Now you may be wondering why I spent the last couple paragraphs talking about myself. Throughout this book I am going to offer advice based on my understanding as someone trained in psychology, but I am also going to draw upon my own personal experiences. Besides, I feel it is important to have a sense of who someone is when you are evaluating their message. As they say, always check your source. If only people on Facebook followed this rule before sharing a political meme . . . oh well, human nature is what it is.

One more thing about me and then we'll move on. After a seminar on happiness one day, an audience member came up to me and said, "So you are happy . . . are you married?" to which I replied, "Of course not, I said I was *happy*."

On more than one occasion, someone implied that my happiness and apparent lack of stress were a function of my being single and childless. Although it is true that I loved being unattached and only responsible for myself, there is a giant pile of research that suggests married people are happier than single people,[6] and people with children are happier than people without[7] (again, remember these are generalizations). Researchers also suggest that one of the primary drivers of happiness is having a sense of purpose.[8] For example, traveling the country helping people can, and does, provide a guy with a healthy dose of purpose. But you know what else works? Being a good partner to someone. Or being a good parent.

My life has changed dramatically since the publication of my last book. My partner, Sarah, and I began seeing each other as I was writing the manuscript. She was working in Colorado for the summer and I was still in Los Angeles trying to be famous. Despite

6   Linda Waite and Maggie Gallagher, *The Case for Marriage: Why Married People are Happier, Healthier and Better Off Financially* (New York, NY: Broadway Books, 2002).

7   Married people, anyway. According to Luis Angeles, "Children and Life Satisfaction," *Journal of Happiness Studies* 11, no. 4 (2010): 523–538.

8   R. W. Robak and P. W. Griffin, "Purpose in life: What is its relationship to happiness, depression, and grieving?" *North American Journal of Psychology* 2, no. 1 (2000): 113–19.

the distance, we felt a connection so strong that we decided to take our relationship to the next level: sell most of our belongings, get rid of our homes, and travel the world together as nomads. You know, like everyone does when they fall in love. A year and a half later we were joined by our beautiful daughter, Alyssa. After continuing to travel for a while, we decided to return to Colorado so I could work on this book. With a partner and a child (holy crap, that's a family!), my life is barely recognizable compared to its previous state.

At the age of forty-five, I became a dad. I know what you are thinking, "Babies having babies! This man is too young to have a child!" No, it's true. I am a father, but honestly, Sarah did most of the work. Forty-five years old and this was my first pregnancy. Well, it was her pregnancy, I just inspired it.

I am older, but I am not that old. One day in Texas, Sarah and I had just finished a speaking engagement and I was standing with Alyssa in my arms greeting members of the audience as they left the room. Sarah was nearby and I mentioned to a woman how lucky I am to be able to take my daughter with me as I tour. She replied, "Yes, and you must love having your grandbaby with you too." The struggle is real, y'all.

And I get it. I have never been more stressed than I am as a parent. My daughter hated me for the first six months of her life because as much as I tried, I simply could not lactate. Whenever I was home alone with her, I was a constant source of disappointment. But beyond being occasionally screamed at, on a daily basis I am concerned about her future, as I hope all parents are for their children. I am frequently plagued by worries about providing for her and doubts about whether I am doing the right thing. She is now eighteen months old and right this moment is trying to pull me away from my computer. Parenthood normally comes with stress, but have you ever tried to write a seventy-thousand-word book while taking care of a demanding toddler?

Seriously, she is tugging on me to go for a walk. Alyssa baby, daddy has to write. I'm on a roll and, . . . well just let me finish this section . . . *okay* I guess we are going outside.

She did, in fact, drag me away from the computer just now. We went to the park down the block and for once I was not the oldest father at the playground, but I was the least tattooed. (Denver is an interesting city.) When we came back, I made us lunch. By the way, I just made my first PB&J as a dad. However, because my kid is only one and a half, I also had to eat it.

I didn't have to share any of that brief departure with you. I could have just put down the computer, gone for a walk, and come home to pick back up where I was, but I did so because it brings me to another point. Besides being a new source of stress, my daughter is also a source of unbelievable happiness for both Sarah and me. All my life, people had been telling me that having children changes everything. "Yeah," I'd reply, "I know. I had a dog."

I had no idea, and there is no way anyone can know, how incredibly gratifying it is to reproduce. Every time I look into my daughter's eyes, my heart melts. Other than crying, everything she does fills me with joy. Just now, she led me to get up, put my shoes on, and head out the door. Leading Sarah and me by the hand is a relatively new behavior for Alyssa. And at the park she tried out some new toys, played with a group of children a bit older than her, and made a new friend. After eating a few bites of her sandwich for lunch, she fell asleep in my arms, so I am now typing this around her. I love watching her learn, grow, and develop. Oh, and when she does cry, I want to do everything in my power to make things better. And because I know that someday she may read this, in case I say differently in the future, every diaper I have ever changed has been an absolute honor (remember that if you ever have to change mine, kid). I never anticipated how much my life would change. Before having a child, I would have never considered sharing a lollipop with another human being.

Sarah and I know plenty of parents who are constantly under stress. We hear from parents of older children all the time about how difficult this period was for them. You know what? Other than a few infrequent situations it has never been that bad for us, and overall it has been spectacular. Parenthood is like any other life event in that how you deal with it influences how it affects you. Before Alyssa, we were both generally positive, resilient people, so it seems reasonable that we would carry those characteristics into this stage of our lives. One thing is certain, I doubt future audience members will suggest that the reason I am so happy and stress-free is my lack of children.

If you read *The Laughing Cure* (and if you haven't, might I suggest adding it to your reading list after this? All proceeds go to keeping a darling baby girl alive), you may remember that one of the benefits of laughter and having a sense of humor is that it helps make us happy. To use a quote often attributed to William James, the father of American psychology, "We don't laugh because we're happy, we're happy because we laugh." Happiness is a great emotion, and really preferable to the alternative, but for many people it is a difficult thing to experience because of stress. If we could just get a handle on stress, we would have greater potential to achieve happiness. Thankfully, laughter and humor also help to reduce stress, which in turn helps makes us happy.[9] As a comedian, and someone who appreciates a good laugh, this is my favorite benefit to mention in my seminars.

For this book, I decided I would focus more heavily on stress management and resilience. I love inspiring happiness in people, and it is important, but good stress management has so many more benefits to our lives than simply making us happy. Stress, as a contributor to so much mental and physical pain, is something that we absolutely need to address.[10] If we could just get people to deal more effectively with stress, we could reduce or even eliminate a great deal of pain and suffering. I do not consider this a self-help book, but rather just some practical advice in dealing with stress presented in a hopefully entertaining way. In this book, I will discuss stress in a bit of detail so that you can understand why it impacts our lives so much. I will also be addressing many of the common questions I receive as a public speaker and expanding

9   I covered this a bit in *The Laughing Cure*, but here are some articles for reference:
    Mary Payne Bennett and Cecile Lengacher, "Humor and Laughter May Influence Health:
    II. Complementary Therapies and Humor in a Clinical Population," *Evidence-Based
    Complementary and Alternative Medicine* 3, no. 2 (June 2006): 187–190.
    Lee S. Berk, Stanley A. Tan, and Dottie Berk, "Cortisol and Catecholamine Stress Hormone
    Decrease is Associated with the Behavior of Perceptual Anticipation of Mirthful Laughter,"
    The FASEB Journal 22, no.1, supplement (March 2008): 946.11–946.11.

10 Including, but not limited to: anxiety, chronic pain, depression, diabetes, fibromyalgia,
    hypertension, immune disorders, obesity, osteoporosis, and so many more!

on the information about stress management I presented in the previous book. As I mentioned earlier, this or any other book is no substitute for professional therapy, so please keep that in mind and seek additional help if you are truly hurting. Stress is a factor in many mental illnesses and disorders,[11] such as depression, anxiety, obsessive-compulsive disorder (OCD), substance use disorder, and of course post-traumatic stress disorder (PTSD), and if you are struggling with these or other issues *please seek out a therapist.* However, reading these pages can potentially help increase your stress-management toolset, and we can all use a little help once in a while. Even those of us who are already happy can benefit, because who can't be happier? It's not like you can max out on happiness.

KEEP IN MIND

- This book is NOT a substitute for therapy in any way.

- This book is ONLY intended for entertainment, information, and advice.

I wrote this book with the general audience in mind, with references for those who would like to seek more information. Even if you are unfamiliar with my style, if you've read this far it should be obvious that this is not an academic or professionally oriented book. I cite a few references but this is far from a proper review of the scientific literature. I provide them as a jumping off point for the curious reader and because I was trained to write for science and old habits die hard. And just in case I get on the

---

11 Actually, with few exceptions, stress is a factor in almost every disorder in the book. That book being: American Psychiatric Association, *Diagnostic and Statistical Manual of Mental Disorders (DSM-5)* (Washington, DC: American Psychiatric Association Publishing, 2013).

Oprah Winfrey Show somehow[12] (maybe she'll return, let's cross our fingers and check under our chairs), keep in mind that some of my stories are exaggerated for effect, but the information I present is true to the best of my knowledge. I may have a fancy degree in psychology, but I am also a comedian. And remember, if you are stressing out about being happy, *you are doing it wrong!*

---

12 I am referring to the controversy around author James Frey and his book *A Million Little Pieces*. If you don't get the reference, don't worry, Sarah didn't get it either.

1

Of Bears and Traffic

Okay, so now that I have properly introduced myself and given you some idea as to where we will be heading in this book, let's start at the beginning, the basics. I know I used the word "stress" a lot in the previous section, but what exactly is it? We all feel stress—we all understand it from an experiential perspective and, in fact, some of us may be feeling it right now—but beyond our experience of it, I think it is important to understand stress in its basic components. The simplest description I have ever come across is that stress is our brain's reaction to a perception of threat. That's it, and that's all.

Notice the mention of threat: that is the key to understanding the response. All stress is a reaction to threat, regardless of whether you are trying to make a deadline, pay a bill, navigate traffic, or fight off an alien invasion. Now, we may not consciously think we are being threatened every time we experience stress, and there may not even be a real threat present, but our brain is reacting as if we are being threatened or are in some sort of danger. Our brain can't tell the difference.

I like to use traffic as an example that helps people understand the source of stress. All of us have been in traffic, probably all of us have gotten stressed out in traffic, so it is a common enough experience. I used to live in Los Angeles, a city famous for its traffic and absolutely nothing else. Think about a time when you were really stressed out in traffic. Maybe it was on your morning commute. Whatever you picture, you might have thought that in that moment the traffic was causing your stress, but unless you live in some *Mad Max*–inspired post-apocalyptic death race world, you were probably wrong.

That traffic was not a threat to you. The cars on that road were not out to get you or attack you in any way. At no point that morning did hundreds of random strangers organize for a meeting and say, "OK, today we are going to make Judy late for work and drive her crazy at the same time! Here's the plan: half of us are going to get in front of her and drive real slow. The other half are going to follow behind her and honk our horns. Now let's do this!" As much as I'd like to see Judy taken down a peg, this did not happen. Also, there is no Judy.

So why did that traffic seem so stressful? Well, our brain creates these things called beliefs, values, and expectations, and they influence how we perceive the world. You may believe that you have to be somewhere at a specific time, say nine in the morning. Maybe your belief is substantiated by others' expectations, because, Judy, we all know you've been warned about showing up to work late. But it is the belief that you are late that is making your brain perceive traffic as a threat to your livelihood. Maybe you value punctuality (unlike Judy) and you think that being late for an appointment reflects negatively on your character. Maybe you simply have an expectation that when you are on a highway you should be driving at a certain speed and the traffic you've encountered this morning contradicts your expectation. Maybe you're just a mess, Judy. Whatever the reason, I would like to point out that in all those scenarios the perceived threat was a product of your thoughts. The traffic was real, but it was your own beliefs, values, and expectations that made the situation into one that you found stressful.

On the other hand, sometimes we are faced with actual threatening situations. The other example I like to use is being attacked by a bear. This is my example of a real source of stress. Just to be clear, I have never been attacked by a bear so even my real example is imaginary. However, I can easily imagine being approached by an angry or defensive bear, fangs exposed, claws outstretched, charging at me and ready to pounce. If we were to ever find ourselves in that situation, the bear would pose a very real and legitimate threat. I believe that if I get into a fistfight with a bear I am going to lose. I expect that if a bear attacks me, it will shred me to pieces, and I value my not being shredded to pieces. My brain would definitely perceive a threat in this situation, and for good reason.

I know there is a chance that some of you may have been attacked by bears, and if this is bringing back horrible memories for you, I'm sorry, but you should have come to terms with that before reading this book. In my public speaking appearances, bears are my go-to animal to make this point. I have tried others, but it just doesn't work well. Playing it safe, I started telling people to imagine they were being attacked by a tiger. I figured, this is North America, what are the odds that someone I was speaking to would have been attacked by a tiger? Tigers don't live here.[13] Then, one day in Louisville (go figure it was in Kentucky), this guy came up to me after the talk and said, "You're not going to believe this, but I was at the zoo one day and the tiger escaped!"[14]

So then I started talking about everyone's favorite imaginary animal, unicorns. The problem with this was that people had a hard time relating to the example. People tend to think of unicorns as nice, benevolent, magical creatures that have glitter in their fur and shoot rainbows out of their butts. Even Judy has a collection of toy unicorns at home. However, a real unicorn will kill you! It has a horn on its head! What do you think that horn is for? That's a weapon for stabbing! It didn't grow that thing so little girls could play ring toss! That unicorn will stab you, stomp all over your body, and shoot rainbows out its butt just to add insult to injury.

---

13 I recently found out that although not wild, an alarming number of privately owned tigers are living in North America. Apparently, they are really easy to buy: Harmon Leon, "America Has a Tiger Problem," *The Observer*, September 11, 2018, https://observer.com/2018/09/america-tiger -problem-buying-big-cats-legal/. *And* crazier still, someone at a Miami high school thought it would be a good idea to have a caged tiger at prom: Kalhan Rosenblatt, "Tiger at Prom? Miami School Faces Backlash for Bringing Exotic Animal to Dance," *NBC News*, May 14, 2018, https://www. nbcnews.com/news/us-news/Miami-school-faces-backlash-bringing-live-tiger-prom-n873846.

14 Thanks to our friends Craig and Nancy, we are staying just a fifteen-minute walk from the Denver Zoo. We bought an annual pass as soon as we arrived and have already been several times. To date there have been no escapes to make my bear example less hypothetical.

You can see why I went back to bears.

Ultimately overcoming stress and managing its impact on our lives depends on this basic realization: most of our stress is from percieved threats, not clear and present threats. If you are going to get all worked up over traffic, consciously or unconsciously, living in the world of what could happen rather than what is happening, you might as well watch out for unicorns.

One of the first pieces of advice I will offer is this: Learn to assess your stress. Learn to tell the difference between bears and traffic. The first thing we should do when we start to feel agitated or stressed is stop and ask ourselves, "Is this situation actually threatening?" If it is, then Houston, we have a probl—uh I mean, bear!

It is a simple question really, and it requires clarity of mind that we often do not have when we are enraged or frightened or whatever, but if we can take a moment to assess our stress it will help us calm down. Imagine again that you are sitting in traffic and you start to feel your blood boil a bit. Before you allow yourself to react, ask yourself if this situation represents an actual threat to you. Chances are, it does not and you will start to calm down.

But what if it *is* threatening? What if you are actually being attacked by a bear? If you answer yes than a follow-up question is in order: "Can I do anything about it?"

The first question is great at helping your rational mind take charge over your stress response (more on this later, I promise) and the second question brings it home to help alter our behavior. Let's break this down in the traffic scenario.

This is me, pretending to be sitting in traffic:

Oh man, this traffic is driving me crazy! I am getting so frustrated! But wait, is this traffic actually threatening? Well, I guess not. Everyone is moving well and nobody is being particularly aggressive, it is just slow. Maybe I should relax and keep my mind off things until it loosens up.

or

Yes, it is a real threat! I have a flight I am trying to catch. If I am late, I could miss it!

In the second scenario, I am understandably stressed. Now can I do anything about it? Realistically the answer is no. I have no ability to magically part the cars in front of me like the Red Sea—I'm no Moses. I'm also not going to convince anyone to move out of my way, and I can't take an alternate route. I'm just going to have to wait it out. Sometimes you just have to sit in traffic.

If you are facing a threatening situation and there is something you can do about it, then you should do that. But if there is nothing you can do about it, what is the point of allowing yourself to get stressed? Now, not only are you going to be late but you have got yourself all worked up with no action to take. You are sitting there just marinating in your own stress. Try not to get any on the seats.

Okay, now let's get attacked by a bear:

Oh no, there is a freaking bear charging toward me!

Yes, but is this situation actually threatening?

Duh, it is a bear! It is most likely going to do some very bad things to me.

Can I do anything about this? Well . . . That's going to depend on a few things, such as what I know about bears, what type of bear is it, what I have in my possession, what is around me, and what kind of physical shape I am in. Let's just say that the answer is "yes." Yes, I believe there is something I can do to help me survive this bear attack. Then I should probably get stressed out.

Does that surprise you? If we are facing an actual threat *and* we can do something about it, our stress response is there to help us out. When we are stressed, our brain and body initiate a series of physiological changes to help us take action against the threat we are facing. When the system works, stress helps increase our chances of survival or catching that flight or meeting that book deadline. Whatever the threat, our experience of stress is there to help us face the challenge.

The problem is that more often than not, there is no bear. Remember, stress is not our reaction to threat, it is our reaction to the perception of threat. If we only felt stressed when we were truly threatened, then stress-related illnesses would be less prevalent than they currently are, and I would not be writing this book.

Thanks to all the generations of humans that lived before us, enduring hardship and creating the modern world, we live really cushy, comfortable lives. When we leave the house, we don't have to be wary of sudden attacks from our enemies, we don't have to compete with other predators for food, and we are rarely, if ever, attacked by bears, or anything else for that matter. We are using a system intended to help us escape bear attacks. Instead, we moan and whine about inconveniences like traffic.

AND NOW FOR THE SKIMMERS:

- When stressed we should ask ourselves, is this an actual threat?

- If it is an actual threat, then can I do anything about it?

Already I believe we have discussed something quite valuable: the need to assess our stressors. Engaging in a little inner dialogue may not seem like a major intervention, but it can be extremely helpful. Let me give you an example of when I had an opportunity to observe this firsthand.

I was giving a seminar on stress, and before we went to a break I gave the audience the same advice I just shared with you. My speaking engagements are usually located in hotel conference centers and most of the time they provide coffee during the breaks. Generally, I use the break time to refill my own cup of coffee as well.

I got into the line, with about two or three women ahead of me. Everything was going smoothly and people were moving along until the woman in front of me made it to the coffee dispenser for her turn. After waiting patiently for those in front of her, she took an empty cup, held it under the spout, and flipped the switch, but no coffee came out. Not a single drop. The woman before her must have gotten the last bit.

I started to notice her reaction to this. Her face became flushed red, she started to shake, and appeared to be visibly upset. Then, she said out loud in a soft voice, "This is not a threat to me," and began to calm down. Here is the thing, she did not know I was standing behind her and at this point I decided to tap her on the shoulder and let her know.

"Finally, somebody gets it!" I said, and we waited for the coffee to be refilled.

What Happens in Our
Head During Stress?

———

Earlier I discussed stress in simple terms using my usual "Bears and Traffic" hypothetical examples. I will let you in on a little secret, for a while I was actually considering "Bears and Traffic" as the title of this book (it sure beats "Untitled Funny Book About How to Cope with Stress"), but I decided against it because I thought it might be misleading for all those readers out there hoping to learn about animals and the cars they drive.

As I mentioned, I use these examples to represent threatening situations, ones where we are probably in some degree of real danger (i.e., bears), and the others where the threat is more likely felt due to our own mental activity or the fact that the dude in front of us is clearly on his cell phone and is driving way too slow to be in the left lane yet he still has his blinker on like he's going to make a left turn. *What is he going to do, drive into oncoming traffic? Who gave this guy a driver's license anyway? Great, now I'm late for my anger management class. Jerk.*

Regardless of how real the stress may or may not be, when our brain perceives a situation as being threatening, the process it engages is the same. Just like airport security, our brain has to take every situation seriously because failure to identify threats could be disastrous. Therefore, whenever we encounter a stimulus, whether it is a bear, a highway full of slow-moving cars, or a traveler who for some reason chose to wear shoes, the first thing our brain has to do is determine if that stimulus is going to kill us. It is a very high-priority decision that the brain has to make before we take any other action. I am sure I don't have to explain to you why it is so important that our brains do this.

Let me pause for a moment to prepare you for the next few paragraphs. As I mentioned in the introduction, this is not a technical book and I do not intend to get into a whole lot of detail; however, I am about to introduce a little about the anatomy of the brain and the nervous system as well as related bodily systems. I feel like I might lose a few of you as you skip ahead, but I promise I will keep it simple and relevant. Besides, a little neuroscientific knowledge never hurt nobody. We all own human brains, so I figure we should have some understanding as to how they work. Plus, my specific area of psychology was neuroscience and "Brain" is even a common misspelling of my first name (even cooler, sometimes they add in my last name and I become "Brain King"), so I feel compelled to discuss the brain. Don't worry (more on that later), this is not a textbook and there will be no exam on Friday.

Getting back into it, the first thing the brain has to do when we encounter a stimulus is determine if it represents a danger. This processing is called threat appraisal, and is carried out by an area of the brain called the amygdala. The amygdala is an almond-shaped bilateral structure located deep in the brain and part of a group of structures known as the limbic system. It is involved in our experience of emotions, learning, memory formation (particularly those relating to emotion), and basic decision-making. I should also point out that the activity of the amygdala, and most of the brain, happens outside of our conscious awareness. That is, this crucial area has an extremely important role in our lives and we are completely oblivious of its activity.

Information about whatever we have encountered is brought into the brain via the sense organs, and is transmitted to the amygdala to be evaluated for potential danger. Contextual details, memories of past experiences, and some instincts factor in to make a quick decision as to whether or not this stimulus is bad news. Say for example we encounter a bear (yes, again). Is that bear bad news—or a *Bad News Bear*? The context could be that we are on a trail all by ourselves deep in the woods of the Sierra Nevada mountains and suddenly realizing that smoked salmon was a bad choice to pack for lunch, or we could be staring the bear down through a fence at the Denver Zoo. Obviously, the context is going to influence our appraisal of threat. Our memories can include direct experiences with bears, but much more likely for most of us it is knowledge we have acquired through indirect means like studying or hearing stories about bear attacks.

Unlike our memories, instincts are not learned, they are inherited as part of our genetic makeup. I am unaware if anyone has been able to identify all our instinctual triggers but I believe that there are certain characteristics common to most predators that we intrinsically respond to, like an arched back, a growl, or exposed teeth. Whatever the threat cues are, it is reasonable to believe they are there. Watching my daughter as she has developed over the past eighteen months has helped confirm this for me. Having no prior knowledge of dogs, the first time she met my brother Jon's dog (a very friendly animal twice her size), she was understandably scared of it.[15] I suspect that in the absence of experience, the amygdala errs on the side of caution, as it damn well should. Her initial fear response was later overcome through repeated exposure and learning, and now like most children her age, she loves dogs (although she seems more comfortable with cats). Most of us, when suddenly facing a bear in our hypothetical situation, would probably have an intrinsic reaction, as I suspect we have zero knowledge of or prior experience with aggressive bears—bear trainers, Jellystone picnickers, and rugged mountain men aside.

The thing about the amygdala is that it is able to process the relevant information extremely fast, especially when compared to other parts of the brain. I mentioned that the amygdala is involved in decision-making, and is an unconscious area of the brain. We also have a conscious part of our brain that we often use to make decisions; in fact you are using it right now to read this sentence. The prefrontal cortex, the part of our brain that sits just behind the forehead, is where most of the activity we refer to as "thinking" occurs. Using this part of our brain to make decisions is completely appropriate most of the time, but it is slow. Our conscious thought process considers the pros and cons of each choice, considers past experiences *and* imagines future outcomes, factors in social norms and expectations, and does a whole bunch of other stuff I am leaving out because this paragraph is already going to be too long, but you get the idea.

---

15 She also had no experience with bears, and the first time she saw a bear on TV in a scene from *Super Troopers 2*, she expressed discomfort and urged me to change the channel.

What Happens in Our Head During Stress?

Conscious decision-making is slow, very slow. Imagine if we engaged that process to decide if we are being threatened. *Is that a bear? I wonder what kind of bear it is. I know that bears can be dangerous, but so can dogs and my brother's dog is really nice. It looks like it could attack, but also maybe it is just curious* . . . and suddenly I am being mauled. We are talking about identifying potential danger here, so the faster we can come to the right conclusion, the more likely we'll survive.

When the amygdala determines that the stimulus represents a potential threat, it sends a signal to an area called the hypothalamus, another part of the limbic system. The hypothalamus in turn activates the sympathetic nervous system, which is responsible for a whole host of physiological changes. These changes, which I will discuss in a later section, all get our body ready for whatever action we will need to take. This entire system works so fast that our body will experience these changes before our conscious mind has caught up. In other words, we will encounter a stimulus, unconsciously decide that it is threatening, and start reacting to it before we are aware of what we've encountered.[16] This is a great thing when we are actually being threatened. For example, before you realize there is a bear, you are likely already reacting to it. However, if the situation does not warrant a stress response, it can cause us to act before we get a chance to think. You could be driving as the traffic suddenly picks up. Before you become aware of it, you are already agitated and that agitation is probably going to influence your behavior.

---

16 This is also what happens when we suffer a panic attack.

Speaking of behavior, our amygdala also sends its information to an area called the nucleus accumbens, located fairly close to the center of the brain. I like to point out its location because if you knew nothing else about it you would probably guess that it's pretty important. With the exception of, say, the Star Destroyer ships from *Star Wars*, generally the more important something is, the more protected it is. Unlike the high-ranking officers of the Empire (whose bridge is located in the most vulnerable part of the ship), not only is the nucleus accumbens protected by the skull but it is also insulated by layers of brain tissue. All the structures packed into the core of the brain are crucial to supporting life. You can live without your ability to think, and a few examples of people that seem to prove this come to mind, but you'd have a hard time living without these areas.

The nucleus accumbens does not produce our behavior, but it is important for motivating it. You may have previously learned that it is involved in our experience of reward, or learning through reinforcement. Those things are true, but to put it simply (my favorite way to put it), the accumbens assesses the relative value of our options. The value of any given option can be positive, as in it is going to improve our life by adding something, commonly pleasurable, to it (we call this "positive reinforcement" or "reward"), or negative, as in it is going to improve our life by removing something uncomfortable or painful (called "negative reinforcement" or "relief"). Basically, I can improve my life by eating chocolate cake or by escaping a threat. The thing about the accumbens is that it doesn't care if life improvement comes from reward or relief, it is the relative

What Happens in Our Head During Stress?

value that matters. If eating cake brings me more immediate value than doing twenty pushups, you can guess which option my brain will pick. I'll have more to say on this later.

Hypothetically, let's say we are facing some sort of threatening situation. Hmmm, I don't know . . . let's say we are being attacked by a bear. Yeah, that's it! Our amygdala has just determined that this situation represents danger and has alerted our sympathetic nervous system. At the same time, it signals our accumbens, which kind of asks itself, "What should I do?" Perhaps it identifies a couple options. Maybe one option is that we can prepare to defend ourselves. Or maybe running is an option, or maybe we can lie down, play dead, and hope the bear is gentle. All of these options involve relief as opposed to reward. I know, it's hard to believe, but there are some problems chocolate cake cannot solve.

Running, preparing for a fight, and playing dead are not very complex behaviors, and that is why they're immediately considered. The nucleus accumbens identifies options that we have practiced so well throughout our lifetime (you know, during all those times you ran, fought, or played dead) that our brain has learned to perform these tasks without thinking about it. Remember that conscious thought in this context would slow us down, so the options are simple well-learned behaviors. You may recognize these three options as fight, flight, or freeze, respectively. Each of these options has a value associated with it based on past experiences, and the option with the greatest relative value is the one your nucleus accumbens is going to pick. Are you a really good fighter? Then pick up a rock or a stick and prepare for battle! Are you a really good runner? Then get those legs moving! Are you like me and really good at neither of those things? I can't even remember the last fight I was in and the last time I ran, I am pretty sure it was to catch an ice cream truck. Better assume the fetal position and hope that you don't taste good. Some of us will even make ourselves not taste good, if you know what I mean, and spoil the meal.[17]

By now you must understand my use of simplified hypothetical examples. But just in case: *do not* take me literally. I am many things, but an expert on bears is not one of them. Before you go boxing ursine beasts or trying to outrun an animal that can reach 40 mph,[18] do a little research. There are resources out there about what to do when you encounter a bear, so don't blame me if you get eaten, Goldilocks.

Let me use another example. Imagine you are driving down the highway and suddenly find yourself in a traffic jam. As soon as your brain picks up on the impending slowdown, your amygdala identifies it as a threat and sends word to your nucleus accumbens. Your accumbens in turn evaluates your options. You can either fight, flee, or freeze. Obviously, these are generic categories of behavior, but how would those options be translated into the traffic situation? Fighting in traffic could mean a number of different behaviors like honking the horn excessively, yelling at other drivers, flipping the bird or flicking them off or whatever you call it locally (pointing at Canada?), or driving aggressively. On the other hand, it is hard to flee from traffic, but maybe you could take the next available exit or even

---

17 Yup, I mean what you are thinking. Loss of bladder control is also common under extreme stress.

18 Assuming you're running from a grizzly.

move over to the shoulder. Let's say that for whatever reason, fighting looks like a more valuable response to your brain than fleeing, and so you start laying into your horn, annoying the inconsiderate drivers who dared to be stuck in traffic before you. I would like to remind you that all of this, from identifying the "threat" of traffic to obnoxiously honking your horn and raising your middle finger, happened without any conscious thought.

At least I like to believe that this behavior is unconsciously motivated; I would have a really low opinion of our species if I didn't. I can't imagine a rational thought process that would lead someone to think this behavior is a potentially useful strategy to cope with traffic. Like we are all going to hear the honking horn and suddenly think, *Hey, I better let this guy through. It sounds like he may be slightly late for work!* It's a fight response, and given the context it may seem perfectly natural to the unconscious brain.

Finally, there is the prefrontal cortex. Not that this completes the entire discussion on brain structures relating to stress, but this is the last one I will bring up. And I already brought it up (you remember that, right?). As I mentioned, the prefrontal cortex is the part of your brain that sits behind your forehead and eye sockets. It is involved in planning, decision-making, problem-solving, attention, and short-term memory. Basically, all the activities we might refer to as "thinking." It is the only part of your brain that you are aware of, therefore I like to refer to it as the home of the conscious mind. It is also the only part of your brain you have direct voluntary control over. You get to decide what types of thoughts you keep in there.

The prefrontal cortex has the ability to override the reactive behaviors I discussed earlier. For example, thanks to your nucleus accumbens you could find yourself sitting in traffic uselessly honking at the person in front of you. You could think to yourself, *Why am I doing this? It is clearly not having the desired effect, I think I'll stop,* and stop honking. You can even ask yourself, *Is this actually a threat to me, and can I do anything about it?*, as I recommended in the last section, which will help you to calm down. You don't even need the inner dialogue, but I'm making a point. Your prefrontal cortex can alter or completely reverse decisions made by other areas of the brain and all you need are your own thoughts. In fact, if you have the right kind of activity in your prefrontal cortex as you enter the traffic, it will prevent your amygdala from identifying it as a threat in the first place.

AGAIN, FOR THOSE READERS WHO ARE JUST FLIPPING THROUGH PAGES:

- We begin responding to stress before we have a chance to think about it.

- However, we have the ability to overcome our initial response.

Unfortunately, a lot of people do not use their conscious mind in the way I just described, and some seem to not use it ... at all. Instead of using our thoughts to modify our behavior, we get caught up in the moment and our stress influences our thoughts. We start to think about how much we hate being in traffic and how that person in front of us has plenty of room to move forward, and *what is the hold up anyway?* Don't these people know that Judy is late for work? Judy has better places to be than in traffic.

Learning how to increase the right kind of prefrontal activity, or thoughts, and being able to consciously redirect choices made by other areas of the brain, is the key to living a less stressful existence.

As I often say: if you don't like the way you feel, change your mind . . . er, thoughts.

Worry Is the Worst

Now that you understand stress as simply a reaction to a perception of threat, I want to share a bit about an interesting phenomenon we all engage in where the brain creates its own stress. I would even argue that the vast majority of the stress we experience is self-induced. That is, we feel stress when there is no real external threat to us, only some challenged belief, value, or expectation of ours. In other words, a thought. Yep, most of our stress is imaginary. Those no-good stinking unicorns.

Worry is a thought process that falls into this category and it is just the *worst*. Worrying is nothing more than internally generated stress—stress we impose on ourselves thanks to some particularly troublesome thoughts. Worrying is a behavior, although a mental one, and we often worry about life stressors, but worry itself can sometimes be the cause of additional stress.

Let me give you an example, again with the traffic. Imagine you get up a little late one morning and hop in the car for your morning commute. On your way to the highway you start thinking about the fact that you woke up later than usual and because of this you might hit additional traffic. You could think to yourself, *Oh man, I bet there is going to be traffic. I am so going to get fired.* Consider what just happened—you are driving normally and you have just caused yourself to elevate your stress level in anticipation of something that hasn't even happened and may not happen. You have generated stress unnecessarily thanks to your own thoughts. And another thing, Judy, you really should get your life together.

I often speak out against worry, and I do so for the reason that it is a really bad habit and one that we may not recognize as such. As a form of mental behavior, worrying too much, over a lifetime, can be a major contributor to developing an emotional disorder like anxiety or even depression. It is a behavior that we can change, and doing so is probably in our best interest.

And yet, we all worry. Maybe not all the time, but we all have moments where our negative anticipations consume us and cause us stress. As I mentioned in my introduction, I am a really happy guy and yet I occasionally worry. I mostly worry about my daughter, like how am I going to provide for her future, am I helping her to grow into a happy and healthy woman, and will she be attacked by bears? Definitely the bear thing. Worrying is a normal activity, which is why it probably doesn't register on anyone's radar when it is problematic. But there are people who worry way too much, about anything and everything. They have practically turned it into a hobby.

One of my college roommates was like that. He was an extreme worrier. Although I eventually earned my doctorate, I was never a traditional college student. For reasons I no longer remember, I dropped out of high school in my senior year, and that sort of thing generally makes it hard to go straight into college (and most drop-outs . . . well, don't). Nobody in my family had been to college, and I didn't exactly hang out with a college-bound group of kids, so I really had no idea what I was doing in the beginning.

I first met my friend James in high school and we actually got our GEDs at the same time. We decided college would be easier if we attempted it together and signed up for a lot of the same classes our first year. We had this one class that met Mondays, Wednesdays, and Fridays. I forget the subject but I remember we had an exam every Friday.

James and I were not the best students (go figure, the bad habits that led us to drop out of high school followed us into college), but we were motivated. One of the major differences between us that I noticed was our approach to those weekly exams. Whereas I would turn in my exam as soon as I finished and duck out of class to get an early start to my weekend, James was the kind of student that wrestled over every question, often second-guessing himself and waiting until the very end of the hour to turn the test in. Later on, we would sometimes meet at the bar on the corner near our apartment. I remember one time in particular when he looked a bit anxious. "Are you okay?" I asked.

"Man, I'm just really worried that I failed that exam," he replied.

"Well, then you probably did," I said. "But worrying about it isn't going to change anything now, you might as well relax and enjoy your Friday night."

I thought it was strange, but he couldn't do that. In fact, all night he kept referencing the class and questions on the exam that he thought he had gotten wrong. He ended up going home early. I woke up the next morning to find that he was already awake and was in the living room with all of his books and notes out, frantically going over them. "Man, you remember that one question? I think I got it wrong." I swear, if he put in this much effort before the exam, he wouldn't have needed to spend his weekend worrying.

But he would worry about it, and all weekend long. On Monday we would get our grades and he would either be pleasantly surprised or have his fears confirmed. Either way it went, his worrying all weekend did absolutely nothing to influence the outcome of the exam. He wasted his weekends, when he could have been wasted. Eventually he decided that college wasn't for him, not because his grades were that bad, but because he couldn't handle the stress.

And that's the thing about worrying, it does nothing to prevent bad things from happening. Worrying does not affect the outcome of a situation, it doesn't make adverse events less likely to occur, it just makes our life less great.

Let me add another step to the advice I gave in the last section. When we start to worry to the point that we start to experience stress, we need to take a moment and ask ourselves, "Can I do anything about this?" If the answer is yes, then do it or make a plan to do it. In fact, if we can do something about a situation and we choose not to for whatever reason, then we are to blame for our own stress. I was once approached by a woman who told me she was really stressed because her best friend had been spreading rumors about her and talking about her behind her back. I said, "Wow . . . you refer to this person as your *best friend*?" Personally, I wouldn't even refer to such a person as a *friend*, let alone give her the *best* spot. But to each their own. She explained that they had known each other for a long time, so that kind of made sense. I asked how long she had known her friend and she said, "About ten years." I then asked how long her friend had been behaving like this, and again she said "About ten years." It was pretty clear to me that this was a problem that could have been solved about ten years ago.

The woman could have broken off the friendship, but what if there isn't anything we can do about our situation? In that case, I think it is helpful to ask ourselves, "If there is nothing I can do about it, then why am I worrying about it?" It is a rhetorical question really, but by thinking that to ourselves, we reduce the likelihood that we will continue thinking about whatever it is that is causing us stress.

My college roommate was unable to see the futility in worrying about an exam he already turned in.

I only recently became a parent, so worrying about children is new to me. I do occasionally worry about my daughter's future, as I previously mentioned, but I try to limit this. I am, however, always concerned for her well-being. Concern, at least the way I use the word, is not the same thing as worry. Both imply a form of caring, but worry can be unnecessary and anxiety inducing: I am concerned for my daughter's life, but I don't worry that she'll be mauled by bears.

I remember once using the aforementioned line of questioning with a friend who was feeling a bit stressed about his kids. First, I asked him what he was worried about. He said, "It's my kids, they are away at college and I'm concerned that they are partying too much instead of studying. I am worried they are going to fail out."

That's a pretty serious concern. I asked him why he thought that. "Well, I keep seeing these pictures they post on Facebook, they are always going to parties and drinking." Let me pause the serious conversation for a minute, because um . . . that is what Facebook is for. You post pictures of yourself partying and having good times with friends. Nobody ever posts a photo of themselves reading a book. You'll never see a post from your kids at home at the dorm, hair messed up, in their pajamas, with the caption, "Hey, guys, this is me studying for an exam!" Social media is for posting pictures of partying. That, and kittens.

"Yeah, I know, but I still can't help worrying about them. They are my kids, you gotta worry about your kids," he said. *Okay*, I thought, and asked him, "Can you do anything about this? "Well, not really. They live in another city." *Okay*, I thought, and asked him, "If you can't do anything about it, then what is the point of worrying about it?"

"Well, they are my kids, you gotta worry about your kids."

"Okay, can you do anything about this?"

"No."

"Okay, if you can't do anything about it, then what is the point of worrying about it?"

"Well, they are my kids . . . "

The conversation cycle continued until, finally, he suggested, "You know, I guess on some level I really just like worrying."

Ladies and gentlemen, we have a breakthrough! I almost never catch that level of self-awareness in people, but he was telling the truth. Some of us enjoy worrying. If it isn't those kids, or the exam, or the potential traffic on our commute, we'll find something else to worry about. If nothing worry-worthy is going on in our immediate lives, we can turn on the news or worry about the things that show up on our Facebook feed.

I love social media, but it really does provide worry fuel for a lot of people. I suspect those same people would worry plenty without it, but at least I wouldn't have to scroll through their alarmist posts to see my friend's vacation pictures. What is interesting to me is that social media is whatever we make it: we control the content we are exposed to.[19] And yet, I often hear from people who quit it because of "all the drama." Which is a shame, because there are so many positive messages being shared on a regular basis. We just have to learn how to filter the nuggets from the dirt.[20]

SPEAKING OF NUGGETS, SKIMMERS, THIS IS FOR YOU:

- If we can't do anything to change a situation, what is the point of worrying about it?

---

19 Although the artificial intelligence algorithms also have an influence, ideally these are supposed to respond to our preferences.

20 So, train them algorithms!

Sometimes people ask me when it is appropriate to worry or if all worrying is stressful. I think these questions are really a case of getting hung up on semantic differences. Realistic concern and worry are not the same thing. There is a big difference between "There might be traffic" and "Oh, man, I am totally going to be late because of traffic." One of them may help you prepare for a situation, the other causes stress. Similarly, there is a difference between understanding that you may encounter bears on your hike through Yosemite National Park and being so worried about bear attacks that you are on edge the entire time, or worse – you don't even go on the hike. Yosemite is one of the most amazing places on Earth. I couldn't imagine being so worried about bears that I would miss out on that experience. By the way, if you haven't been, and you have the means, then definitely go! The views are breathtaking, and chances are you'll recognize it from the Ansel Adams poster that was hanging in your friend's dorm room. I try to visit at least once a year.[21]

I frequently ask people to tell me why they worry, and I hardly ever get the answer I am after. For example, I just shared a conversation with a worrying friend in which I asked him why he worried and he said that he thought his kids were partying too much while away at college. Like most people whom I ask, he was telling me what he worries about, not why he worries. If you are a worrier, why do you worry? Understanding why you repeatedly engage in this behavior could be a great help in overcoming it.

---

21 It is such a beautiful place that on several occasions I have brought friends there for their first time. For example, when I found out my friend, comedian and radio host Paul Brumbaugh, had never been, despite living his entire life within four hours away, I insisted on taking him.

In the interest of full disclosure and as you may have figured out by now, I am not a worrier. So I can't speak on the impulse to worry from my personal experience; however, it's pretty clear to me that nobody seems to consciously decide to worry. I doubt anyone ever says to themselves, "Hey, you know I really feel like worrying right now. Let's see, what should I worry about? I know, I'll worry about those kids!" In other words, it does not appear to be a behavior initiated by the conscious mind, or the prefrontal cortex. Therefore, it is probably selected unconsciously by the nucleus accumbens in its basic decision-making.

As you now know, decisions made by the accumbens are the result of comparing the relative benefit of whatever options are currently being presented. Because we know the brain chose to worry—it is an observed behavior—that must mean that the action of worrying was associated with a greater potential value than any of its competitors. That also means that worrying apparently has value to the brain. Now, what are the benefits of worrying?

You may recall that the benefit of an action is that it either provides some sort of reward or it provides relief. So the benefits of worry have to fall into one of those two options. We can probably rule out reward, or positive reinforcement. I am sure that nobody derives pleasure from worrying. At least I have never heard anyone say something like "Oh, man, last night I was worrying *so* good!" or "I can't wait to get home from work so I can worry some more!" or even "I've got a whole bunch of things I'm going to worry about this weekend, it is going to be awesome. You should come over!" No, I have never been invited to a worry party (and I would totally go just for . . . science), so I am pretty sure worry is not a pleasurable activity. And if worry isn't providing the brain with some reward, then it must provide relief. But relief from what?

That is a hard question for most people to answer, so here is where the doctorate in psychology comes in handy. As it turns out, worry provides relief to the brain for a very uncomfortable condition it sometimes experiences called "inactivity." The brain is a vast electrical circuit comprised of individual cells called "neurons" making connections to one another. Neurons are specialized cells that conduct electricity, and they are regularly transmitting electrical impulses to each other via their connections. Networks of connected cells stimulating each other can, and do, represent everything in your head, from the definition of the word "twerk," to a memory of when you first learned how to twerk, the instructions on how to make that booty twerk, and everything else related to twerking or otherwise that you store up there.

Stimulating those neurons also lets the brain know that a particular connection is still relevant to your life. However, under-stimulated connections are probably no longer relevant and if they are under-stimulated long enough, they can be lost. Therefore, an inactive connection is one that may not exist in the future, and an inactive network is at risk as well. Without regular activity, parts of our brain are at risk. You have probably heard the phrase, "Use it or lose it"—well, there is a reason you forgot most of what you learned in college (it was actually your Ansel Adams poster). The brain does not like to be inactive.

So now you can imagine that inactivity is an uncomfortable condition for the brain. You may not experience this condition as uncomfortable, you might just label it as boredom. Usually, the outside world provides the brain with plenty of stimulation, but sometimes it does not and the brain has to stimulate itself. Worry is one way that the brain can generate its own activity. Yes, worry relieves boredom. And I believe this is why most worrying occurs.

Think about it. If you are a worrier, when do you worry? You probably don't worry when your brain is actively engaged in some task. You probably don't worry when you are focused on an activity, deep in thought, or being thoroughly entertained. More than likely, you worry when you have time on your hands or when your brain is not otherwise occupied. You worry to relieve boredom, which should be no surprise, as boredom already motivates a lot of behavior that people would prefer to change. People eat when they are bored. People drink when they are bored. Some people smoke to give their brains and hands something to do. Some people pick fights, get angry, or just stir things up. And some people worry. In other words, you worry to give your brain something to do. It probably doesn't matter if it's the kids, the economy, or something on the news, if you are a worrier and your brain is in need of some activity, you will find something to worry about.

So now that you (hopefully) understand why you worry, what can you do about it? In the simplest terms, changing a behavior usually involves understanding why you do it and finding a suitable alternative. Because worrying relieves inactivity by giving the brain something to do, if you want to worry less you should find something else for your brain to do. But then what could possibly be a suitable alternative to worrying? How about literally anything else!

When you feel the onset of worrisome thoughts, understand that your brain needs some of that sweet, sweet activity and give it some. Read a book. Take a walk. Do the dishes. Clean the living room. Watch a good TV show. Start a conversation with someone (just don't talk about the thing you are worried about). Anything, literally *anything*! To overcome worry you have to redirect your train of thoughts. Change the channel in your brain.

In most cases, a simple distraction can be exactly what we need. Distraction is even a common practice in therapy. Whenever Sarah, a therapist, has a patient who is ruminating so much that they are having a hard time focusing on therapy, she finds some way to redirect their thoughts by changing the subject to something positive. She'll start talking with them about their grandchildren or their favorite music, and it helps take their mind off their worries for a moment. She does the same with our daughter—whenever Alyssa is upset, Sarah is really good at refocusing her attention to help her calm down.

Redirecting your brain may sound easy to do, and relatively speaking it is, but it requires awareness. The problem many of us have is that once we start worrying, those thoughts consume us and we just keep fueling the fire with more. But, if we have enough awareness to realize that we are heading down that path, we can consciously interrupt the flow by introducing an alternate route. When my mind starts to be dominated by stress, I like to take a drive. I find that driving helps me calm down and gather my thoughts. You may find something else works for you, as long as you are changing the channel.

AND SKIMMERS, HERE YOU GO:

- Learning to keep our brain active can help us avoid excessive worrying.

It is hard to stop worrying. But the good thing is that at least you have options. You have a lot of options. There is practically no limit to what you can do to satisfy your brain's need for activity as an alternative to worrying. Unfortunately, too often the behavior we desire to change has few, if any, suitable alternatives, like worrying has. In those cases, we just have to find a way to manage life without, and that is super tough. For example, my brain loves when I eat ice cream and loves to dish out cravings for it. Now, let me ask you, what could possibly be a suitable alternative to eating ice cream? I'll give you a hint, there is no alternative to ice cream! The pleasure my brain receives from my eating ice cream is not matched by my eating any other substance (don't even try to convince me that Froyo tastes basically the same). When my brain wants ice cream the only thing that will satisfy it is ice cream.[22] What am I going to do, eat kale? Even kale-flavored ice cream is gross. If I want to overcome my love of ice cream, I have to learn how to live without it. And that is no easy task, because even lactose intolerance fails to convince my brain that eating ice cream is any less awesome. Worrying may be a tough behavior to overcome, but at least you have plenty of alternatives.

I should also note that not everyone worries when their brain needs something to do. People also have positive responses to boredom as well. Some people exercise. Some people, myself included, daydream or do something creative. When my mind wanders, I sometimes come up with jokes. If Sarah is with me, I'll

---

22 My daughter seems to agree with me. On a recent outing for lunch I may have accidentally mentioned ice cream in the car, but when I got to the drive-through, I was told the machine was down. I got her a cookie instead, and she threw it on the floor.

test them out on her and if she laughs they might make it into my comedy act. I have been known to spontaneously write poetry or make up song lyrics, not that any of those are ever any good (Sarah can attest to that), but these are some of the activities that give my brain something to do when it's bored.

What Happens to Our Bodies During Stress?

I first met my partner, Sarah, in Gainesville, Florida. I was touring through the state doing seminars on stress or happiness or whatever, and she was one of a few hundred people who saw me on that stop. She is an occupational therapist, and was attending to gain some insight that might help her with her clients. A few years later, we had a baby. I think she got her money's worth.

Sarah is beautiful, intelligent, kind, and funny. (Of course she is, how else could she have landed this prize of a man?) She is also very happy, healthy, and extremely resilient. However, sometimes, even the best of us go through a rough period. She often tells the story about a few years before we met, when she went to see a doctor for an annual physical. All of her test results, blood values, and body weight were within normal limits. On paper she was perfectly healthy. However, at the time she had been having some general pain issues, including her joints and in one shoulder. She was also suffering from frequent migraines.

Her doctor looked at everything; she asked Sarah about her lifestyle and in particular about her home life, work, and daily commute. She suspected that there must be something that Sarah was doing at that point in her life that was causing these issues. Perhaps something was causing stress that was leading to these issues. The doctor said, "If you stop to think about it, I bet you know exactly what it is." It took Sarah less than two seconds to identify the source of her stress.

Several months before, Sarah had taken a contract job to work at a facility over an hour away from her home; some days she spent up to three hours commuting through traffic. She reported to a difficult boss, a micromanager type, who, by constantly checking up on Sarah's work, made her feel as if she wasn't doing her job. She also received no recognition for exceptional work, or praise when praise was due. For example, she once saved the life of a client using CPR, an act that several nurses at the facility felt was commendable enough to tell her boss about. And ... nothing. Not even a pat on the back.

Realizing that the stress was affecting her health, Sarah put in her notice immediately. To help survive her remaining time, she started practicing breathing exercises and power poses at the start of her shift, and made a point to leave the building to take a walk at lunch. After work hours, she danced tango a lot more than she had been. At home, she spent more time outside on her porch, writing, and working in her garden. Finally, after her last day on the job, she starting working a job much closer to home—literally two minutes from home—and also started her own business. Her symptoms went away.

Similarly, I don't remember exactly when my left eye started twitching, it just appeared and gradually got worse and worse. Like Sarah's health issues, it happened during a particularly tough time in my life. I was working at a job I hated and living in an apartment I could barely afford. I never complained about it or even sought a professional opinion on my eye twitch. Not because I was against going to a doctor, but I had more pressing issues occupying my attention. Also, just as Sarah had experienced, my symptom went away after I experienced some changes in my life. Unlike Sarah, my relief came from being laid off. I didn't realize it then, but getting fired from that position was just what the doctor ordered.

Prolonged exposure to stress can have a negative impact on our physical health and general well-being. Also, stress can affect individuals differently. Sarah suffered bodily pain and headaches from stress; I experienced involuntary muscle spasms in my eyelids (and probably some additional symptoms I was too stressed to notice). But why? As I described earlier, stress is our brain's reaction to a percieved threat. Why would our response to threat cause us pain and other problems?

Before I get into that, let me first discuss some of the physical effects of stress. Previously I mentioned how the amygdala, after identifying something as threatening, sends signals via the hypothalamus to activate the sympathetic nervous system. Man, that's a lot of anatomical terms for one sentence. I'm not sure how technical I can get without turning this into a textbook. Sarah just convinced me that most people have probably heard of this stuff, so I'll keep it. This is a network of nerves that connect the spinal cord to many bodily organs and when activated, it is responsible for most of the physiological changes that occur. Our eyes dilate, our heart rate increases. Stress can cause us to perspire or cease digestion, and can inhibit erections in males. It makes us sweaty, bloated, and limp.

The sympathetic nervous system also triggers the adrenal glands to start producing adrenaline, that sweet hormone sought by bungee jumpers and extreme sports enthusiasts. Basically, anyone who owns a GoPro. Adrenaline surges through our body and energizes us. It increases blood flow to the muscles, blood sugar, and the force and frequency of our high fives with our bros. Adrenaline is also released during stress, but we generally don't think of it as a stress hormone. That honorable distinction goes to cortisol.

When the hypothalamus receives the stress signal from the amygdala, it activates the sympathetic nervous system as I have just described, and also stimulates the release of a hormone called ACTH into the bloodstream.[23] This hormone travels through the arteries down to the adrenal glands and tells them to start cranking out cortisol because something nasty is about to hit the fan. Like adrenaline, cortisol also increases our blood sugar and has a lot of additional effects on the body. The adrenaline and cortisol, now surging through our body, are delivered to our organs faster thanks to the increased heart rate.

Whether mediated by the sympathetic nervous system or cir-culating hormones, all of these changes that take place in our body

---

23 Adrenocorticotropic hormone (ACTH). I'm simplifying here of course; in slightly more detail, the hypothalamus actually produces a hormone called corticotropin releasing factor (CRF), which in turn stimulates ACTH secretion from the pituitary gland.

are supposed to be beneficial. They serve to increase our energy and make our body more efficient, two things that may prove to be quite helpful if we are being attacked by a bear. We are mobilized for some form of action, and that action is going to be fight, flight, or freeze. We are going to defend ourselves or attack in some way, flee or try to escape, or in some scenarios we will do nothing.

Most people are familiar with the standard "fight or flight" dichotomy, and really that is probably all we need to understand, but I like to throw in "freeze" because it is a common behavioral reaction. Think about how many times you may have been so overwhelmed with stress that you became incredibly inactive. Maybe you were sitting at your desk at work, handed an incredibly daunting task with an unrealistic deadline, and instead of diving right in and tackling that bad boy (fight), or asking your boss for an extension or help (flight), you just sat there unable to do anything (freeze). I've been there. Remember the job that made my eye twitch?

It is easy to understand freezing in the bear attack scenario. A lot of people will freeze up when overcome with fear. Even the Black Panther froze (and his sister made fun of him for it) despite the fact that he has super powers *and* advanced technology![24] Marvel movies aside, my favorite "freeze" story took place during my time in graduate school.

I had a friend who was given a car by her family. The problem was, it had a standard transmission and she didn't know how to drive a stick. What a great gift! "Here: it's a car that you can't

---

24 As his bodyguard, Okoye, said, he froze "Like an antelope in headlights" in *Black Panther* (Atlanta, GA: Marvel Studios, 2018).

drive!" Being one of her few friends who knew how to drive manual, I offered to teach her. We started off in the parking lot and I explained how the clutch pedal worked, when to press it down, and how to shift gears. Then she practiced a bit. Of course, there were some initial stalls, but after a few minutes she got the hang of it and was shifting all the way up to third gear. I asked if she was ready to hit the streets and she said yes. We left campus, drove a few blocks, and everything seemed fine. We caught a red light, and she slowed down to a stop without incident. She was a little stressed, elevated heart rate and all, but not out of control.

At a four-way intersection, we were the first car in our lane at the light. As soon as the light turned green, she went to press the gas pedal but did something wrong and the car stalled. Now, in traffic we have cars coming at us from the opposite direction and cars coming up from behind and she freezes. In this context freezing meant letting go of the steering wheel, lifting her feet off the pedals, and *covering her eyes!* She yelled, "I can't take this" and threw her arm across her face.

Suddenly, I too became stressed. My fight response kicked in and from the passenger's seat I grabbed the wheel, stretched my leg over the center console to work the pedals, and steered us out of traffic. Nobody was hurt and after we calmed down, we had a good laugh about the whole thing. You know, the whole thing where we could have been seriously injured.

I didn't realize until much later that her reaction, which I had trouble understanding at the time, was a common response to stress. Remember how I discussed how the brain picks actions based on whichever one has the most potential value given our previous experiences? I believe that if neither option looks appealing, the brain will choose to freeze or do nothing. In the case of a bear attack, for example, successfully fighting off or running from a bear are extremely unlikely outcomes for most people. In the absence of a good option, many people would choose to freeze. Similarly, at that moment sitting in the car in the middle of the intersection, my friend was faced with a choice. In a car, both fight and flight require driving skills, and to a brain that lacks confidence in its ability to drive neither option will likely hold much value . . . so she froze.

Ever have so much to do that you can't seem to get out of bed? I've been there.

I will admit that freezing probably does not require an increase in energy so we are safe usually just focusing on fight vs. flight, but it is interesting.

Now let me get back to why our stress response would cause Sarah to suffer body pain and make my eye twitch. One of the things about our fight or flight response is that it represents a short-term solution to a short-term problem. Danger in nature is usually temporary and if we are successful, it should be resolved quickly. Do you know the nice thing about being attacked by a bear? It doesn't last very long. One way or another, that bear attack is going to be over fast.

Elevating our blood sugar or heart rate temporarily so that we can increase our chances of survival is not a bad thing; in fact, stress works toward our advantage during these moments. However, you can imagine that maintaining a high level of blood sugar for an extended period of time can have a negative impact on our health. Similarly, long-term elevation of our heart rate can also cause complications. Unfortunately, most of the stress we experience is not due to actual danger, but perceived threats that have a tendency to linger around. I don't know how long Sarah was stuck at her difficult contract, but even if she was only contracted for six months, those were six months of feeling on edge. Six months of sitting in traffic every day. Six months of unnecessarily elevated adrenaline and cortisol. Prolonged exposure to stress can, and does, take its toll. My eye-twitch job lasted about a year.

There are other downsides to long-term exposure, not from what stress increases but from what it suppresses. After countless generations over the entire span of evolutionary history, there is a wisdom to our stress response. Our body has a limited amount of resources, whether it is water, sugar for energy, or different proteins, neurotransmitters, and hormones. Having finite resources means our body has to give consideration to how it distributes them, like during World War II, when the government rationed food, fuel, and materials like rubber and steel to support the war effort. If our body is under attack, then it needs all available resources to survive that attack. That means cutting off any irrelevant systems.

What is irrelevant when we are stressed? Well, if we think about this in terms of being attacked by a bear, we can identify a few things. For example, our immune system is not necessary. If we are being attacked, what difference does it make if we catch a cold? *Sure, that bear seems dangerous, but I should probably get this cough checked out.* Our digestive system can definitely be sacrificed. If we have any food in our stomach, we can probably wait to digest it (or just get rid of it altogether), and if we are being attacked by a bear, we probably don't want to stop to make a sandwich. Healing from wounds or injuries and repairing the cells of our body are not priorities either. Sure, it is important for our long-term health, but if we don't survive this current situation there may not *be* a long term. For that matter, growing and developing our body isn't important either. Sex drive is definitely not important. What is the point of reproduction when you are being attacked by a bear? In fact, if you do feel like reproducing when being attacked by a bear … man, that's an unfortunate fetish.[25]

Part of the problem is the simplicity of our body's stress response. We have lots of different types of stressors, but just a single response system. From your body's perspective it doesn't matter if you are being attacked by a bear or have an annoying boss, the response is the same. One of those situations is life-threatening and surviving it demands a lot from the body, the other … doesn't. It is probably not necessary to shut off your immune system or suppress your sex drive because your boss is a dick. The response is overkill, and yet that is what we are working with.

AND FOR THE SKIMMERS:

- Prolonged exposure to stress can contribute to a wide variety of physical illnesses.

_____

25 Unless you find a partner with a good costume.

Stress contributes to a whole lot of physical conditions that we suffer, not just high blood pressure and diabetes. This is why long-term exposure to stress can make people take longer to recover from illness or heal from wounds. This is why we sometimes have stomach cramps or get nauseous. And this is why we may sometimes experience migraine headaches, bodily pain, or twitchy eyes.

Negative Emotions and the Stress That Inspires Them

As I mentioned, I am writing this in Colorado. It is early October, and yesterday, without warning, the weather turned from fairly moderate to full-on winter. My friends tell me it just does that here, but it caught us off guard. Sure, we knew winter was coming, but we thought we had a few more weeks before we would be bulking up with layers. So, earlier this evening Sarah and I were out at a shopping center in Denver picking up a few things. This being the period just before Halloween, there was a lot of fun stuff for sale, in addition to the more sensible things we were looking for. The candy, though, we walked by quickly. We are handing out bitcoins to the trick-or-treaters. Let's see if that joke is still relevant by the time this book is published.[26]

---

26 Who am I kidding, it's barely relevant now. The Facebook post of this joke only garnished a mediocre thirteen likes.

I love Halloween. I love dressing up, I love haunted houses, corn mazes, crazy Halloween parties—it really is one of my favorite times of the year. All holidays are great, but I really love the party ones: Halloween, New Year's, Mardi Gras, Arbor Day . . . (man, them trees sure know how to let loose!). This year is going to be a little different, because this will be my daughter's first time trick-or-treating, and as you might imagine I am a little excited about it. Anyway, while shopping I saw a few Halloween costumes that would just look adorable on our little girl, but Sarah, being the more sensible of the two of us, kept us focused on our objective and vetoed my costume purchase. I don't remember what I said, but I was a bit irritated. "You're hangry," she said. It was true, I had skipped lunch and as we walked into the store, I was feeling a bit of the old hunger pangs.

Have you ever been hangry? I imagine it is a common experience, common enough that the word isn't triggering my spell-check at the moment. We sometimes get a little irritated when we haven't eaten, or haven't eaten enough. Hunger is a physical state that can influence our emotions. Hunger and stress are very closely related. I would even suggest that we could think of hunger as a type of stress. From your body's perspective, hunger certainly threatens its continued existence.

As with being hangry, one of the reasons that stress has such a huge impact on our lives is that it has a direct influence on our emotional state. You might remember that I quoted William James in the introduction. James is referred to as the father of American psychology, and his work was extensive. To this day, we still teach

Negative Emotions and the Stress That Inspires Them

about and refer to his theories—well, at least I know I do. I talk about him all the time; in fact, I just talked about him earlier today and I am about to do it again. One of his theories I find most helpful is the James-Lange Theory of Emotion.[27]

To put it simply, we feel emotions because of our brain's interpretation of our physiological state. Whenever we encounter a stimulus, like a bear or finding ourselves suddenly sitting in traffic, our body reacts by triggering some familiar physiological changes. Unless you are one of those readers whom I suspect skipped the discussion on the brain, you already have an understanding of the mechanisms behind this, the amygdala and sympathetic nervous system. Our heart rate might increase and we might start to perspire. James then suggested that our brain, receiving feedback from the body, interprets the physiological condition in the context of what is going on at the moment. On some level, the brain is putting the information together that 1) there is a bear charging toward me; and 2) my heart rate is elevated (among other things), therefore I must be afraid. And just like that I am overcome with the emotion of fear.

Now, let's consider why we have emotions in the first place. Emotions influence behavior, specifically by helping us react in a manner that is appropriate for the moment. Think about all the diverse behaviors that a human brain is capable of producing. From playing a piano and dribbling a basketball, to computing mathematics and writing a book, each one of us is capable of a tremendous variety of potential behaviors (albeit, not to the same

---

27 Walter B. Cannon, "The James-Lange Theory of Emotions: A Critical Examination and an Alternative Theory," *American Journal of Psychology* 39 (January 1927): 106–124.

level of proficiency). Not all of those behaviors are appropriate for the situation we find ourselves in. Emotions help restrict our options so we are more likely to choose a behavior that is right for us. For example, imagine again that we are being attacked by a bear. Whenever I visualize this example, I always imagine that the bear is about thirty yards away, running toward me. In that moment, you don't want to suddenly feel inspired to write a poem ("Ah, the duality of nature, so beautiful and yet so fierce"). No, you don't want to do that. You also don't want to see that bear and think, *You know that reminds me, my mother-in-law is visiting this weekend. I should really clean the bathroom.* You don't want to entertain thoughts like that. You definitely don't want to think, *You know, with that bear chasing me this would make a really great selfie.* It would be the last selfie you ever took. It seems obvious to us, but without the emotion of fear, your brain might just wander into some inappropriate territory like that. You want your brain to be fully focused on surviving that bear encounter.

Fear is a negative emotion, and given this perspective, we can see how fear is an emotional response to stress. However, it is not our only possible response. The context of the moment also includes our own thoughts, and depending on what we are thinking we may react differently. We could add it all together as I did above and perhaps conclude, *I am afraid of that bear.* A simple, and probably a common, reaction. We could even go a different direction, wondering, *How dare that bear threaten me?! The nerve of this bear, does that bear know who I am?* and get mad. Or, we could even think to ourselves, *Oh man, why do bears always attack me? That's three times this week! What is it about me that makes bears want to attack me all the time?* and feel saddened by the encounter. The point that I am making is that fear, anger, and sadness are all negative emotions and can all be caused by stress.

Emotions help restrict the range of potential behaviors our brain will consider. All of them do this to us, even the positive ones. Take love, for example. I'm referring to the passionate love we feel in the early stages of a relationship, not the more companionate style of love that we develop over time where it's like, "Yes, I love you, but I want to sleep in separate rooms." Think about the last time you fell in love and how in the early stages thoughts of that person interfered with your ability and motivation to perform other tasks. The last time I felt that way was when Sarah and I first started dating (how crazy would it be if I gave a different example?). I was in Los Angeles writing my last book; she was in Colorado on a therapy contract. It was a long-distance relationship, but neither of us is a stranger to travel and every weekend one of us would visit the other. When we weren't together, we were on the phone. It would be an understatement to say that this had an impact on the pace of my writing. Negative emotions may have an even stronger impact on our behavior. Have you ever known someone with depression? One of the most difficult symptoms of depression isn't feeling sad, it is feeling unmotivated. Anxiety has a similar impact on our behavior.

You may recall from the previous section that there are three basic categories of behavioral reactions to threat: fight, flight, or freeze. If we interpret our physiology as the emotion of fear, we increase the likelihood we will attempt to flee or escape. If we interpret our physiology as anger, we increase our chances of attempting to fight. Finally, if we interpret our physiology as sadness, we may be more likely to freeze or do nothing.

IN OTHER WORDS:

- Stress influences our emotions, and in turn our response to stress is influenced by our emotions.

Just as hunger can sometimes lead to crankiness (spell-check recognizes "hanger" but still seems to take issue with "hungappy"), stress can lead to negative emotions.

Some people like to differentiate types of stress, stating that so-called good stress helps energize us to get the job done, meet a challenge, or overcome an obstacle. On the other hand, bad stress causes us pain and misfortune. However, remember that the function of *all* stress, good or bad, is to help us overcome or escape threat. As far as I am aware, all stress has the same effect on the body. It increases our energy, elevates our heart rate, and pumps the hormones adrenaline and cortisol through our veins. If I get stressed in traffic, all those physiological changes amount to squat as they don't help me in the slightest. Unless I can take a different route, I can't do anything to change my situation while in traffic, so now I'm just sitting there with an elevating heart rate, marinating in my own cortisol. That's not good meat. I would argue that stress in this context is not very functional. On the other hand, if I am being attacked by an unfriendly Goldilocks hater, then that increased energy and heart rate just might help me enhance my chances of survival. In that case, the stress would be very functional.

Consider that whenever we activate our stress response, functional or not, we are inhibiting our immune system and preventing our body from being able to heal.

In my opinion, stress that serves a purpose, whether it is surviving a bear or meeting a deadline, is a good *use* of stress. It should be understood that stress, good or bad, has the same impact on the body regardless of how it is used. If our stress causes our heart rate to elevate, and in turn increases our risk for stress-related health problems, we should make it count. Don't get stressed over the piddly, inconsequential events that seem to plague us on a regular basis. In other words, only get stressed when you are faced with a "bear."

SKIMMERS, TAKE NOTE:

- Our stress response should be engaged only when it can help us.

Nobody can tell you what your bears are. Only *you* can decide what is worth stressing over. If you think traffic is worth it, then fine. Feel free to get stressed in traffic every day, twice a day. You know, whatever makes you happy. Personally, I don't think traffic is worth stressing over—if I'm late then I'm going to be late. The things that I consider bears include direct threats to my safety and well-being, and the safety and well-being of my loved ones; threats to my livelihood and again those of my loved ones; and maybe threats to valued property. Also, anything that makes my daughter unhappy, because yes, being a parent does introduce new stress into my life.

Regardless of what you consider worth stressing over, one thing is clear: not everything is worth it. If you struggle with stress and are interested in reducing it, then keep reading.

2

―――――

Making Decisions Under Fire

If you don't mind, I would like to get personal for a minute. This is something that I have been holding in my entire life, but now with the publication of this book I would like to set the record straight: I love chocolate. Wow, it feels so good to open up like this. I know most of us like chocolate, but for me I think it goes beyond that. Not that I eat it all the time, but if I see it or smell it, then I crave it. And I'm going to get it. Even if it isn't mine. Man, I am getting hungry just thinking about it now.

Have you ever seen those king-sized candy bars? Maybe *you* can avoid them but my last name is King. They were made specifically for me. When you open the package, you find out it is actually split into two smaller candy bars. On the package it reads something like, "Enjoy one half now, save half for later!" I have *never* saved half for later. I cannot even comprehend doing so. How can you leave an unfinished candy bar? I have noticed the same thing with bags of M&M's, not the giant bags you buy to fill candy dishes, but the larger-than-normal-sized bags you see hanging at the convenience store. The bags are resealable, you know, in case you don't finish the whole bag. To me, that is just a waste of a seal mechanism.

Some might describe their love of chocolate by saying they are a "chocoholic," but I really don't like that term. First of all, there is no such thing as "chocohol" and "-aholic" is not a suffix. You can't just add that to some noun and pretend like it makes sense. "But Brian, what about me? I'm a shopaholic!" No, you just really like shopping. "But I'm a workaholic!" No, you just really hate your family.

I am being nitpicky here, but that is what comedians do. I don't really care if you choose to describe yourself as a chocoholic, shopaholic, workaholic, or anything-aholic. I know what you mean. I don't like using those terms because I don't think they are fair to alcoholics. It just isn't a comparable experience. My struggle with chocolate is no way as severe as an alcoholic's struggle with alcohol. I have never once woken up in a stranger's bed because they had Hershey's . . . Okay, well there was this one time.

Another thing about me, I consume quite a bit of coffee. I am not sure how I compare to most coffee drinkers, but compared to nondrinkers, I am a total lush. A "coffee-aholic" if you will. On the road I am a frequent customer of Starbucks. I do like, and sometimes prefer, independent shops, but the convenience of having Starbucks locations everywhere just works out well. Plus, Sarah and I rack up the points for free drinks on their loyalty program.

No other coffee chain caters to the touring life as well as Starbucks.

Starbucks has an amazing chocolate chunk cookie. I honestly think it is one of the best cookies I've ever had. The chocolate-to-cookie dough ratio is perfect; it is always chewy and it is thick so there is some substance when you bite into it. They keep it on display right by the cash register too, tempting me with a good time. But as much as I enjoy their cookie, I am watching my calorie intake and I try to pass it up whenever I get my caffeine fix. My nucleus accumbens must believe there is a lot of value in that cookie, because nearly every time I finish ordering the barista will ask me, "Would you like something else?" and I have to consciously hold back the words, "I'll take one of those chocolate chunk cookies please." If I am not careful, I will order a cookie automatically before I get a chance to realize it. That is under normal, relaxed conditions. If I am stressed, you better believe I am leaving that store with a cookie.

But why? Aside from momentarily making me feel better by providing me with pleasure, eating that cookie does absolutely nothing to eliminate my stress. Unless by some very rare chance I was actually stressing out about the lack of delicious chocolate chunk cookies in my belly, cookie consumption is entirely unrelated to whatever it is that has me worked up. Let's say, hypothetically, that I am trying to write a book and take care of my one-and-a-half-year-old daughter during the day. Suppose, again this is completely hypothetical, that for the past few days the daughter I love so much has been making it impossible to get anything done. Imagine in this hypothetical situation that I decided to take my daughter on a walk down Colfax Avenue and stumbled into a

Starbucks. Now, sitting with a mouth full of cookie, I still haven't made any progress on my book. Hypothetically.

Have you ever noticed that stress has a tendency to bring out our so-called "bad habits"? Whatever behavior you are actively trying to suppress or change, your inclination to do so seems to materialize immediately during a period of stress. People smoke when they are stressed, drink alcohol, use drugs, eat, or even worry and ruminate on negative thoughts. There is something about stress that brings out the behaviors we are trying to avoid. I use eating chocolate as a common, relatable example, but understand that it can be anything. Whatever behavior your nucleus accumbens thinks is the best option in a given situation has an increased likelihood of being expressed. It isn't my fault that I went off my diet, my nucleus accumbens just thinks chocolate is awesome (unfortunately, my prefrontal cortex agrees).

You may recall that earlier I explained that when we are under stress our nucleus accumbens evaluates the relative value of our current behavioral options and picks the best one. I should also mention that the nucleus accumbens is doing this all the time, not just when we are under stress. Every moment of our lives our brain is analyzing and deciding which behaviors are in our best interest. We aren't aware of any of this activity because it occurs outside of our prefrontal cortex, but it helps motivate our behavior, and influences our consciously chosen behavior as well.

Imagine a situation where the accumbens determines that two possible actions have about the same potential value. It is like the Coke vs. Pepsi dilemma. For most people, those two options are nearly identical and are basically interchangeable (unlike left and right Twix, where one is very clearly better than the other). Some people have a strong preference, but most of us really don't care whether we drink Coke or Pepsi as they both satisfy the same basic craving. Well, what if our survival of a threatening situation depended on making the right choice? Our brain would have to have a mechanism to force a choice, and it does.

I am not going to go into too much detail here (slightly more in the footnotes).[28] However, when we are stressed and facing multiple options, any small advantage that one has over the other is amplified to help the accumbens decide. Suppose we are generally indifferent about Coke or Pepsi, but we have slightly better past experiences with Coke. That little bit of edge becomes amplified when we are stressed, increasing the likelihood that we will go with our favorite. This is an adaptive mechanism that helps our brain make a tough choice under pressure. If running and fighting are relatively similar in their potential value, but one has a slight advantage over the other, this mechanism helps make sure we pick our best possible option, even when our conscious mind would say, "Ah, whatever."

This means that when we are in a stressed state and navigating through the world, any time we encounter an opportunity to do something our brain prefers, we are more likely to do it. It probably has absolutely nothing to do with alleviating our stress, but the brain doesn't know that. All it knows is that we are stressed and that a chocolate chunk cookie would taste really damn good right about now.

---

28 When the hypothalamus produces CRF, that hormone in turn activates an area called the dorsal raphe nucleus. This structure has widespread connections in the brain and in the accumbens helps increase the difference between choices.

- Not only can stress negatively affect our health, it can also lead to unhealthy behaviors.

Note though that stress does not solely catalyze unhealthy behaviors. If I had lived life differently and trained my brain to really enjoy jogging, then under stress I would be more likely to go for a jog. Too bad I never learned to like jogging.

The morning after writing that last section I drove down to Colorado Springs for a book signing at a Barnes & Noble. I try to do as many book signings as I can fit into my schedule and now that we are in Denver for a few months, my schedule has some openings. Since the publication of my last book, I have learned that being a successful author, much like being a successful comedian, takes a lot of work. Books by famous people sell themselves, but nobody is waiting in line for my new release (yet). To give you an idea of what I am talking about, the morning of the signing a woman came up to my table and said, "I've never heard of you." So, I answered, "That's why I'm here. Have you heard of J. K. Rowling?" "Oh yes!" she said, to which I replied, "That's why she's not here." Maybe I would see more success if I wrote about teenage wizards or vampires in high school, or got on a hit TV show, but until then I am happy to travel the world and promote my work as much as possible.

When I do signings like this one, I do not get compensated by the bookstore, my publisher, or anyone really. This is just the state of the industry, and not at all a statement about Barnes & Noble or my publishers. To give you an idea of what an author is up against,

I asked another man if he would like to check out my book. He replied, "I don't read." (He certainly picked the right place to spend his Saturday afternoon.) I wish these were isolated interactions, but they play out almost daily. The struggle is real, folks. No, I do not expect compensation. I do these events solely because I want people to read my books and I am grateful for the opportunities.

However, a lot of Barnes & Noble locations have a Starbucks inside of them, and frequently they will offer me a complimentary coffee drink, as they did in Colorado Springs. I thanked them and went to the counter to place my order. As I was checking out, the barista asked me if I would like anything else and out popped those all-too-familiar words: "Yes, I'll have one of those chocolate chunk cookies, please." I finished my order and while waiting for my coffee wondered why I let my guard down.

Sometimes life imitates art.

I wasn't very hungry. In fact, we stopped for lunch on our drive down. The mindless inclination to order a cookie was so strange to me because I literally wrote about this exact subject the night before and here it was, playing out just as I had described it. Was I stressed? I did not feel stressed—but sometimes, especially in long-term situations, we adapt, and the stressed state begins to feel normal. I have been working hard on this book, sequestering myself at home with Alyssa during the day, and staying in to edit at night. It is hard to get a lot done while she is awake, but thankfully she usually passes out around nine. (Some people just can't hold their liquor.) Writing is a voluntary exercise, but I do have a deadline and required word count. Could I possibly be stressed about writing a book about coping with stress?

And just then I remembered something that makes me happier than chocolate: getting things for free.

- There ain't nothing wrong with a free cookie.

It's Never Too Late to Change

Sarah and I have been traveling together for over three years, and we use a wide variety of accommodations depending on our circumstances. If we are traveling for a speaking event or a comedy gig, we usually stay in the hotel provided by the organizer or venue. This means that occasionally we get to stay in some really awesome resorts well outside of our means. When we are responsible for our own expenses, we try to stick with a modest budget. Both of us have become experts in finding great travel deals. We stay with friends and family whenever we can, not just to save money, but because it gives us an opportunity to spend time with the people we care about. For longer stays, furnished apartments listed on websites like Airbnb are ideal.[29]

We recently spent a few of months in Montreal, Quebec, and found an awesome apartment on Airbnb. It belonged to a couple

---

29 Like any service, before you book an Airbnb check out what you are signing up for. Although mostly great, we have had some bad experiences too.

that were planning a vacation to Europe at the same time we were to be in Canada, so it worked out really well. They must have been music lovers because among the usual furnishings was a piano. Sarah had always wanted to learn how to play, and taking this as an opportunity, she found a teacher and signed up for lessons. She practiced every week we were in town, which was challenging as Alyssa also seemed to want to bang the piano keys each session. In a short time, Sarah has gotten pretty good and continues to practice whenever she gets the chance, which is difficult with a small child around.

It will be a while before Sarah is composing her own sonatas, but I can't wait until that sweet, sweet sonata money starts rolling in! Sarah and I are people who are always pursuing new interests and learning new things. While she was learning piano, I was learning how to tolerate listening to the scales over and over and over without wanting to go too far in with the Q-tip.

If someone were to image Sarah's brain after several months of practice with the piano, they would probably see a few changes reflecting her newly acquired skill. This change is something we refer to as "neuroplasticity." It refers to the fact that our brains are capable of structurally changing in order to keep up with the demands of our lives. The science is relatively new, but since about the 1960s, researchers have been increasing our understanding of how the brain changes and its capacity to do so. The mechanisms involved are quite complicated, and I will spare you the details in the interest of keeping this from reading like a textbook.

However, I do want to point out that our brain has the capacity to change. This is significant because for the longest time, we thought it didn't. I am a few decades younger than the initial studies of neuroplasticity, and yet I remember being taught in college that during our developmental years our brain was coming together to help shape the kind of adult we would be and once the human brain got to the age of maturity, around the early twenties, it no longer had the ability to change. I was taught this, I believed this, and I taught this to others. Most people do not see a lot of significant change to their brain over the course of their adult life, so it seemed to make sense even though we were wrong.

Imagine that, for whatever reason, you have gone through life training your brain to overreact to adverse situations. Or, maybe you have taught yourself to worry unnecessarily or ruminate on negative thoughts. Maybe your brain has learned to make you lay on the horn whenever you find yourself in traffic. The nice thing about neuroplasticity research is that it shows that whatever behavior you wish to change about yourself, you have the capacity to do so. This is why therapy works.

Don't misunderstand: just because we can change, doesn't mean we will change. In a previous section I discussed how my brain loves chocolate so much that I sometimes order cookies without thinking about it, and how it is too bad my brain never learned to like jogging. Guess how many times I have gone jogging since writing that sentence? If you guessed anything above zero you are incredibly optimistic, and I thank you, but unfortunately you are wrong. Now guess how many cookies I have eaten in that time frame? Shut up. Keep your answer to yourself! Change is really hard, and I suspect this is one reason why we thought the adult brain lacked the ability to do so. We are notoriously inept when it comes to changing our behavior. Our brain gets used to the tried-and-true behaviors that served us well in the past, and is often resistant to putting forth the effort to acquire new ones. This is why we need therapy.

Sarah had to force herself to sit down at that piano and practice hitting those keys. She had to find times when Alyssa was asleep, occupied, or on a walk with daddy to do so. I am sure there were plenty of days when she would rather have enjoyed a nice sit on the couch or some mindless TV watching, but she made a point to keep up her practice. Her weekly lessons with her teacher gave her incentive to practice and each week she would come home with new assignments to work on. Just like in therapy.

I don't play piano, but learning to do so has got to be easier than many of the behavioral changes most of us try to make, like quitting smoking, managing our tempers, or exercising; however, Sarah's piano education still requires perseverance and dedication. Yes, I would imagine that it is harder to quit worrying, or to quit getting angry all the time. Yet, just as people can learn how to play the piano, people can learn to cope with and manage behaviors related to stress. Science shows that we have the capacity for change, it is just really hard. Like jogging.

I hope this doesn't discourage anyone from trying to improve themselves, but the reality is that change is difficult, and most of us are not successful in our attempts. But, unless there are some special circumstances, like brain damage for example, changing our behavior is not impossible. I like to point that out because maybe knowing this will help some of us to keep trying. We may attempt to change some aspect of our behavior and fail, but if we keep practicing, eventually we can get there.

- It is never too late to change how we cope with stress.

Interestingly enough, one thing that interferes with our brain's ability to change is stress. Stress decreases the production of a hormone called brain-derived neurotrophic factor, or BDNF, which is needed for neuroplasticity. Even more reason to learn how to get a handle on it.

Crawling Up That Step

I never really thought much about having children, as I found joy in other things in my life. Plus, I was extremely immature. (Well, that much hasn't changed, but now I have a kid.) One reason I'm glad that I waited until later in my life to have a child is that I think I might be in a better position to notice her development, having studied psychology for so long, and I'm aware of things about her that I may not have picked up on when I was younger.

For example, I remember the time she encountered the step connecting my parents' sunken living room with the rest of the house. We were visiting for a week and Alyssa was still just crawling to get around. On one of the first days, I watched as she noticed the step and crawled up to it. She didn't know what to make of it, and crawled away discouraged. The next day she again crawled up to it but this time threw her leg up on it. She was still unsuccessful in overcoming this hurdle, but she tried again the next day. Finally, after a few days of trial runs, I watched her crawl right up to that step, over it, and continue into the rest of the house like a pro. One small step for a baby, one giant step in making daddy proud. Next, she'll be training for the Olympics.

Every parent has moments like that, but what occurred to me was how resilient she was after her initial setback. Unlike some adults, she did not sit around feeling sorry for herself after her first failed attempt. She did not seem angry, frustrated, or sad, and I am pretty sure she did not consider herself a failure. Instead, she moved on from the event and went back to it with a new plan of attack. It was a thrill to watch her set a goal for herself, learn from her failed attempts, and ultimately triumph.

Earlier today Alyssa got to choose an item from her basket of Halloween candy. Honestly, I am amazed she has any left but she has done a great job saving it. She picked a Tootsie Roll, and held it in her hand as we walked to the car. Once we were all strapped up inside, Sarah turned around to help her unwrap it and we found her sitting with a mouthful of Tootsie, minus a wrapper. At first, we were concerned that she may have swallowed it, but there it was lying on the floor of the car. At just over eighteen months our daughter had figured out how to unwrap her own candy! That's not exactly a milestone behavior, but at this age all challenges are opportunities to learn, and the look of pride on her face as she was chomping down on paperless candy of her own doing was priceless. I am a proud daddy. My little girl is smart.

Not too long ago I spent a few years touring the country and discussing the importance of psychological resilience, particularly as it pertains to stress. Resilience is our ability to recover from adversity, to bounce back or return to equilibrium after experiencing an adverse event. It is a major component in coping with and recovering from stressful events. Watching my little girl tackle that step or figuring out how to unwrap her own candy, I realized that, right in front of me, was an excellent model of resilience. Children are naturally resilient; it is part of the job of being a kid. Unfortunately, resilience is a trait that I believe some of us lose as we grow older.

Most adults face greater challenges than having to crawl up a step, but her perseverance, her refusal to get frustrated, and her reluctance to give up are all characteristic of being resilient.

Recovery time following an adverse event is often used as a measure of resilience.[30] Bad things happen all the time, and to all of us. Think about this: in general when something bad happens, how quickly do you bounce back? Do you get over it relatively soon or does the negative emotion tend to linger around? People who recover faster are more resilient, whereas people who tend to take a bit longer are less resilient. Obviously, what is considered a healthy recovery period is going to vary depending on the nature of the event. Some things are going to require more time than others. Let me give you a recent example.

Every time I have a public appearance, whether it is a speaking engagement, a comedy show, or a book signing, I always make sure I have a pen in my pocket for signing autographs. I never really buy pens, I just kind of "acquire" them, but there is a particular type of

---

30 Not that I do that much research in this area, but my preferred definition and measure of resilience is from: Richard J. Davidson and Sharon Begley, *The Emotional Life of Your Brain* (New York: Hudson Street Press, 2012).

pen that I prefer over all others. I don't know the brand, but it fits my hand perfectly. The ink flows consistently and leaves a great solid line every time I use it. It's my favorite pen and whenever I have one, I try to hold onto it and keep it in my jacket pocket. Recently I did a book signing and when the first person asked me for an autograph, I reached into my jacket pocket and my pen was not there. I had lost my favorite pen—and I was devastated! I had to settle for using a cheap ballpoint pen and I was really bummed for the rest of the event. Just kidding, I had almost no reaction because it is just a stupid pen. Sure, I liked it, but it was a trivial possession and not worth any degree of negative reaction.

But people frequently overreact to the loss of such meaningless items. Obviously, a loss of a pen would be an event most of us would recover quickly from, but a more severe event is going to take some time to get over. Still, some of us will recover faster than others. Resilience is our metaphorical ability to take an emotional punch.

I love movies, particularly big budget action, special-effects–heavy movies. They are really the only ones that I bother to see in the theater anymore. Also, the industry is dominated by movies based on the comic books I loved as a nerdy teenager, and now, as a nerdy adult, I enjoy watching these characters come alive on the big screen. If you aren't a superhero movie geek, you won't know that there is a scene in the first Captain America[31] movie where a short and scrawny Steve Rogers (the man who would later be injected with the super soldier serum to give him the body of actor

---

31 Of course, I am talking about the 2011 film: *Captain America: The First Avenger,* directed by Joe Johnston (United States: Paramount Pictures, 2011), Motion Picture.

Chris Evans) is at a theater. When a man heckles the program during a World War II newsreel, patriotic Steve asks him to shut up. The next scene cuts to the much larger heckler now beating the crap out of Steve in an alley. He punches him straight in the face, each time knocking him down, and each time Steve Rogers gets up. After the third punch the man says, "You just don't know when to give up do you?" to which Steve replies, "I can do this all day." That response could be stubbornness, but I like to think of it as resilience.

Resilience has been shown to be a function of the prefrontal cortex, which I previously mentioned is the part of the brain that we think with.[32] Put simply, our thoughts make us resilient. How we process information and what we think following an adverse event has a great deal of influence over how quickly we will recover. Remember that the prefrontal cortex has the ability to override activity from other areas of the brain and our thoughts influence our emotional and physiological reactions. Imagine if I had reacted to losing my pen by throwing a fit and dwelling on how special, how perfect, how irreplaceable it was. You know, really exaggerating the sense of loss. I would probably be affected by the situation at least for a bit longer.

When my daughter was crawling up that step, she did not yet have any language skills, so I can only imagine what her inner thoughts might have been. However, based on her actions they were most likely not discouraging. She also smiled a lot, which is normal for

---

32 Davidson and Begley, *The Emotional Life of Your Brain.*

her. This gives me another clue into what could have been going on inside her head as she tackled that challenge.

Psychological resilience is very strongly associated with happiness. If you are happy, you are managing your stress well, and if you are stressed you are probably not happy. It is hard to imagine being stressed and happy at the same time. Both experiences are functions of activity in the prefrontal cortex. However, it isn't activity in the entire prefrontal cortex that relates to these experiences, but rather when there is more activity on the left side than the right side. When there is more left activity than right activity, people report feeling happy and appear calm. When there is more activity on the right than left, people report feeling stressed, anxious, and worried. In other words, the thoughts that help you cope with stress are the same thoughts that make you happy. Conversely, thoughts that make you happy help suppress stress. Earlier I mentioned that if we have the right kind of activity in the prefrontal cortex as we enter traffic, it can prevent our brains from feeling threatened in the first place.

There is evidence that happiness and resilience are partially genetic.[33] Feeling happy or stressed are temporary states that come and go, but overall each of us has a general level of happiness. For example, I am typically quite happy, but I don't think anyone would ever describe me as "cheerful" or "bubbly." I know people who are like that, and I believe they are naturally way happier than I am. I also know people who, regardless of circumstance, never seem to be all that happy. You may be familiar with the old "nature vs. nurture" debate. That is, the debate over which factor shapes

---

33 Lyubomirsky, *The How of Happiness.*

a person more: biology or environment. The debate is not really much of a debate at all, as most researchers agree both are important to shaping our psychology. When it comes to happiness, the genetic component is thought to be half. Fifty percent of how happy you are right now is attributed to your genes, about 10 percent is due to your circumstances, and the rest to your behaviors and thoughts.[34] Happiness and resilience may be partially genetic, but we have a lot of potential to modify our emotional state.

AND NOW FOR THE SKIMMERS:

- Psychological resilience is our ability to overcome a challenge, to bounce back after an adverse event, or to cope with stress.

- Resilience is highly related to happiness, and both are functions of how we think about the events we experience.

- Skimming is the best way to read a book. Totes.

---

34 Lyubomirsky, *The How of Happiness.*

3

Having Goals and Making Plans

As long as I can remember, I have always been less affected by stress than those around me. I remember keeping calm in cars full of screaming kids, not getting worked up over setbacks, and just keeping my cool in situations where others seemed to lose it. I remember first learning the definition of "lackadaisical" when a teacher used it to describe my apparent lack of worry about something that was most likely really, really important.[35] For what it was worth, I always seemed to share my outlook with others whenever possible.

For example, when I was in college at the University of Texas at Austin, I went to the campus store to buy a new computer. Upon learning my name, the student technician that was assisting me said, "Brian King? I once worked with a guy named Brian King."

---

35 Sarcasm. Duh.

We figured out that at one point a few years earlier, we were both working at the same Taco Bell location. I didn't remember him, but he clearly knew who I was.

Have you ever worked fast food? I spent my first few years out of high school working wherever I could. I stuffed tacos and burritos, I flipped and flame-broiled burgers, I even cooked and delivered pizzas. Generally speaking, working in fast food can be extremely stressful. The pace is relentless, there is almost always a line of customers inside the store and in the drive-through, and all expect fast service. When things slowed down, management pressured us to look busy even if we weren't. It was not unusual for me to be pushing a broom across a perfectly clean floor because there was literally nothing else to do. Not to mention that all of this activity was typically carried out in a steamy hot kitchen while wearing some form of polyester uniform. I made $3.35 an hour and was grateful for it. Not a lot of doors swing wide open for high school dropouts. I worked with an interesting assortment of retirees, ex-convicts, current convicts on work release, and general unemployables, and occasionally there was a high school or college student. The computer technician was one of those students.

As he was going over the details of my new computer, the technician told me that the reason he remembered my name was because of something I had said to him. One day, during a particularly tough shift, he was feeling a bit overwhelmed balancing work with school. Apparently, I said something like, "Don't worry about it, it's just Taco Bell,"[36] and reminded him to keep his eyes on the bigger

---

36 Not that there is anything wrong with that. Despite working there for nearly a year, to this day it remains my favorite fast food.

picture, like that sweet student technician job waiting for him in the near future. Honestly, I have no idea what I said to him after "it's just Taco Bell," but whatever I said stuck in this guy's head long enough that he thanked me for my advice years later. He had momentarily lost sight of his long-term goal in the midst of taco stress.

Having something to look forward to can really help us endure a lot. Yeah, those jobs were stressful. School was stressful. Hell, life was stressful. At one point during this period of my life, I was essentially homeless. I slept bottom bunk with my best friend above me at his family's trailer in the country. The few belongings I had were stored in another friend's garage. I worked a series of low-wage jobs and took classes at the community college, but I never let it get to me. I find it funny that when I meet people now, they know me as an educated comedian/speaker with a loving partner and an incredible kid. When I talk about handling stress, it's because I have handled some stress.

There were a few things I can identify that helped me keep my composure during that time in my life. First, I had a goal that I was working toward. College gave me a sense of purpose and, as I have since learned in researching happiness and resilience, having a sense of purpose goes a very long way. As long as I knew I was making progress on my education, I felt I could endure anything life threw at me. Second, I was resourceful. When my car broke down and I could not afford to get it fixed, I did my class readings on my bus commute. Luckily, when I briefly became homeless, my friend's parents offered me their home, but I had a plan to sleep on campus in all-night study halls and shower at the gym if they hadn't. As long as I cleaned up, wore a backpack, and looked like a student, I imagined it would be pretty easy to get by on a large university campus. I never had to put this plan into action, but just imagining that I had a possible solution helped me cope. Third, I knew that if things truly got unbearable, I had a safety net. At any time, my parents would have welcomed me back into their home. My strong sense of purpose, willingness to use the resources available to me, and having a plan for the worst-case scenario kept me from feeling all that stressed out throughout a very stressful time. Again, every single one of these components—goal pursuit, problem-solving, and planning for contingencies—are functions of reasoning.

Resilient people approach life by thinking and planning; they see their problems or adverse events as temporary and/or solvable. That was definitely the case for me in my early college years—I felt that my situation was temporary and under control. And, in my case, it was.

To this day, my response to most stressful situations is to problem solve and develop a plan or two. Recently, while on tour, Sarah and I ran into a potential snag. We were in Jacksonville, Florida, with both of our cars and needed to pick up a rental from the airport, to which we would return after three weeks. We parked one of our cars at the airport, and to save money we parked our other car with a friend of Sarah's who had an empty space in her driveway. Everything went according to plan—we dropped off my Mustang at the friend's house, drove Sarah's Prius to the airport, picked up our rental, and were on our way to Tennessee.

We toured all across that state, from Memphis (famous for Elvis) to Johnson City (famous for, I don't know . . . Johnson?)

then made our way back to Florida for a series of Panhandle gigs before coming into Gainesville almost two weeks later, where we got a call from Sarah's friend. "I have to schedule a delivery, and I may need to have your car towed." What the hell? Setting aside the strange logic, we were now in a situation where I realized we left our car with someone whose first impulse was to have it towed the moment it posed an inconvenience. Towing and impound fees are not cheap, plus I really like my Mustang, so this was kind of a bear. Immediately I began working on a plan. We had one more gig in Daytona Beach before we were to fly to New York, so in the worst-case scenario one of us (Sarah) could drive up to Jacksonville in the rental, meet another friend of ours to help drive the Mustang to another parking spot, then drive back to Daytona Beach before the end of the gig and our flight. It would suck, but it was doable. Thankfully, a simple phone call to Sarah's friend solved the problem, but if it hadn't, we had a plan.

Remember what I discussed earlier: negative emotion can interfere with our ability to think by restricting the range of options that we will consider. Sometimes being able to come up with a good plan requires creative thought, and is better accomplished when we are calm and thinking clearly.

Resilience is a state of mind, an attitude. Just to be clear, resilient people are not in denial. When the problem feels out of control, they get stressed. It just might take a bit longer and a much greater threat to push them over the edge. In other words, they will stress about bears but probably feel fine in traffic. When I try to explain the resilient attitude to less resilient people, inevitably phrases like "relax" or "no worries" or "take it easy" will pop out of my mouth. As in, "Relax, it's no big deal, just take it easy." In fact, I can relate to the Eagles song "Take It Easy" because it, or at least the chorus, is about resilience.[37]

> Take it easy, take it easy
> Don't let the sound of your own wheels drive you crazy
> Lighten up while you still can
> Don't even try to understand
> Just find a place to make your stand, and take it easy

I'm no music expert, but that song would have probably been a lot less successful if it was called "Just Be Resilient." On another note, how cool would it have been if that last line went "Just take a minute to make a plan, then take it easy?"

I bet nobody is suddenly comforted when told to just relax or take it easy in the midst of a full-on episode. Telling someone who is enraged, anxious, or hopeless to just relax could be perceived as dismissive at best, and at worst could stress them even further. Depending on the situation, I usually try to validate the person's feelings instead.

I was once driving somewhere in the Australian Outback when a car flew past me with its driver angrily honking the horn. I don't know why he honked—maybe I was going too slow, maybe I swerved to avoid a kangaroo or something[38]—but whatever the reason, I found myself in an encounter with the driver at the next

---

37 More so than say, "Desperado."

38 Seriously, they are like deer out there.

gas station.[39] I barely had a chance to get out of my car, before an angry British woman was berating me in the language they invented. She yelled, "That was very dangerous what you did back there! My husband had to swerve around you!" Again, I had zero idea what she was talking about, but British anger is the worst kind of anger, so I simply said, "I'm sorry, it's a good thing he was able to do that!" and she just kind of looked at me, confused, and went inside the store. Perhaps she was disappointed that I did not join her in an argument. The time to develop our stress-management skills is not when we are jacked up full of cortisol, that's when we need to exercise them. We need to work on our problem-solving, planning, and other positive cognitive activities before we find ourselves facing that bear. Otherwise, the sound of our own wheels just might drive us somewhere we don't want to go.

Feeling in Control, Even When We're Not

About a year after Sarah and I started touring together we took a summer trip to Montreal. We were originally planning on an extended trip to London, England, but somehow forgot to

---

39 In the Outback, as with most of Australia, you never want to pass up a gas station.

reserve our flights and by the time we were looking to take off, airfare was prohibitively expensive. Because we still had the time off and wanted to leave the country, we decided to head north to Canada. We eventually drove across the Trans-Canada Highway, but first spent a few weeks in Montreal. I had been several times, but this was Sarah's first visit. We loved it. Montreal is a striking city, vibrant and alive, with a European flavor thanks to its French culture. We had such a great time that when we left one of us was pregnant. I'll let you guess which one.

The following year, with Alyssa barely a few months old, we decided to go back to Montreal, this time spending our whole summer there. We still loved it, although no new babies were produced this time (that I know of). Instead, we decided to purchase a home. We met a wonderful real estate agent, Raymond LaRivière, and spent a week shopping before putting a bid down on a beautiful condo. It was accepted and a couple of weeks later we were homeowners. Two days after finalizing the purchase, we left town to begin our new seminar tour back in the US. We never even got to spend a night in our new place.

Because we had work in the United States, we left Canada and listed the condo for rent. We hired Raymond and his company to find us some tenants, but this was autumn and winter in Quebec, and from what we hear, it gets cold there. Really cold. A few months went by and our condo sat empty, which was concerning but not too stressful. Thankfully, they found a couple from New Brunswick that wanted to rent our space as a weekend getaway spot. You would think that would have provided us with a bit of relief, but that was when the real stress kicked in.

As soon as our tenants moved in, they reported an odor that was so foul they ended up spending the night in a hotel. Sarah and I were in Florida working on a contract at the time, and were very surprised to learn that our tenants were unhappy and that our beloved condo was home to some mysterious funk. Our home inspection gave us no reason for concern, and for the entire time it was on the market no one had reported anything wrong. Our agent scheduled a few tests, and a possible sewer leak was discovered under our kitchen. We were lucky that our tenants were only planning on living there part-time because our cabinets and appliances had to be removed and the entire kitchen floor was going to have to be dug out to find the leak. Hearing this news, seeing the photos, and receiving angry emails in French all contributed to elevating my stress levels much higher than they have been in years. Visions of Tom Hanks and Shelley Long in the movie *The Money Pit* entered my head as I tried to figure out how to transfer my savings to Canada.

I joke about being an older father, but this was my first home purchase, so that makes two counts toward a delayed adulthood. At forty-five, I finally did something most people do a decade younger.[40] Although, I imagine that most people do not buy their first home in a foreign country where they do not reside and do not speak the official language, but hey, that's just how I roll. Not too many people drop out of high school to wind up getting a doctorate either. Homeownership can be stressful for anyone, but I was starting to think that perhaps I had made a serious mistake.

---

40 According to the annual survey conducted by the National Association of Realtors, because yes, I totally looked this up.

It was one thing after another and, though I will spare you the gory details, ultimately the ordeal spread out over a couple of months. The entire time, Sarah and I were fifteen hundred miles away and helpless to do anything. I was plagued with negative thoughts; I worried about the condo daily and imagined my investment literally flushing down the Montreal sewer system. Sarah had previously owned a home so she was a little less affected, but my stress response was fully engaged. As I previously mentioned, I love social media but I rarely use it to vent negativity. During this time in my life I found it really difficult to remain positive. I remember my friend Frank sent me an encouraging message. He said, "You got this." But that was precisely the problem, I didn't "got this." We had to put our trust in people in Montreal and hope that everything was taken care of. Not that we knew what to do, but the worst part of it all was that we were not present to do anything about it.

Other than having a checkbook, I felt completely powerless. I had no control.

If you'll bear with me, let's return to bears. Once again, imagine an aggressive behemoth bolting toward you. That is a naturally stressful situation. Now imagine that you are not just standing there, but you are holding a loaded tranquilizer gun. Suddenly the situation as described becomes a lot less distressing: you have the ability to solve that problem. Similarly, imagine that bear is running toward you but instead of just standing there helpless, you are sitting in a Jeep and when it gets too close for comfort you just have to hit the gas. Either way, you feel as if you have some influence over the outcome. You feel as if you have some control.

Resilient people approach their problems as if they are sitting in a Jeep holding a tranquilizer gun. The brain has connections between the prefrontal cortex and other areas that mediate the stress response, which effectively allows the conscious mind to shut off the stress response.[41] It is as if the brain, after assessing the level of potential threat it is facing, suddenly says to itself: "I got this." When you feel like a problem is something that you can handle, it no longer causes you stress. Again, resilience is an attitude.

It is worth noting too that when we feel in control, all of the negative effects of stress are reduced or eliminated. Feeling stressed is really feeling out of control, to put it very simply. Every stressful situation is really just a situation where the brain does not feel it has any control. Think about being in traffic, a situation where we have very little control. Think about being attacked by a bear—if you ever find yourself in such a situation, I am willing to bet that the bear is in control. Think about work. Your boss or whatever authority you have to answer to is in control. People worry about world events, potential disasters, economic forces, political changes, being victimized, busted sewer pipes under their newly purchased Montreal condos, and all sorts of other things that they have no control over.

Feeling in control is not the same thing as being controlling. People that are controlling are annoying. They are the worst kind of people, and if you are one of them let me just say on behalf of your family, friends, and coworkers, knock it off. It is also not the same thing as being in control. We can feel as if we have some ability to influence the outcome of a situation, even when other

---

41 Amy F. T. Arnsten, "Stress Signaling Pathways that Impair Prefrontal Cortex Structure and Function," *Nature Reviews Neuroscience* 10, no. 6 (June 2009): 410–422.

factors also have some influence. The more we feel as if we have influence, the more stress we can handle.

In most situations, I have a strong sense of control. The Montreal condo problem was really tough for me because I am so used to feeling in control, and I had none. Ultimately everything worked out fine, and through it all Sarah and I became close friends with Raymond, who really went way beyond the call of duty to help us. So if you are in the market for property in Montreal, I know a guy.[42]

We all feel in control over some situations in our life, and we all have our breaking point. I refer to our stress threshold as the point at which we stop feeling as if we *got this* and start feeling a bit overwhelmed. I also refer to our stress tolerance as the amount of stress we can handle before being pushed over the edge. Resilience is not an either/or type of construct, but rather one that varies along a spectrum. We all have a limit to what we can handle, but some of us have a higher limit than others.

Whenever I think about people on the high end of the resiliency spectrum, I always think about people who work in law enforcement or are in the military, or are professional hitmen. Not that I have ever known a professional hitman, but I bet that is a job that requires an awfully high tolerance for stress. However, I have known many police officers and members of the military, and they do seem to be able to handle a lot of stress on, and off, the job. Having been raised in a military household, I have spent

---

42 I can't recommend him enough; if you find yourself interested in a home in Montreal, particularly in Le Plateau-Mont-Royal, look for Raymond LaRivière on signs everywhere or at www.raymondlariviere.com.

Feeling in Control, Even When We're Not

a lot of time in the city of Fayetteville, North Carolina, which is home to the Army's Fort Bragg. Fort Bragg is notable because by population it is the largest military installation in the entire world; it is the location of the United States Army Special Operations Command headquarters; and it is home to the 82nd Airborne Division, a special breed of badass.

I imagine there aren't too many jobs as potentially stressful as that of an Army paratrooper. Imagine that your job description included flying into the air and jumping out of a perfectly good airplane on a regular basis. Now imagine that job, only this time imagine that your boss not only wants you to jump out of the airplane but wants you to land in an area where people want to kill you. *Hey, you see that camp down there? The one full of angry dudes with guns? Yeah, try to land near that.* That is an enormous amount of potential threat, and I think I would lose my damn mind in that situation. However, there are plenty of men and women in our society who seem to be able to perform these functions just fine. I know there have to be personality factors that contribute to their success, but I suspect a lot of it comes from a sense of control developed through their training. When you are jumping out of an airplane, you are not in control (the wind and this invisible force called gravity are in control), but, with knowledge and experience, you know that there is something you can do to influence the outcome of the situation.

The military, the police force, and related professions include occupations with a high degree of risk, and therefore it takes individuals with a high tolerance for stress to be successful. On the other hand, there is the low end of the spectrum. No job groups come to mind at this end, but I imagine people at the low end of the spectrum to be the kinds of people who are really negatively affected by traffic. Sure, we all have our moments, but for some people the stress of their daily commute can be a significant problem. We don't all have to jump out of airplanes, but most of us do have to navigate traffic.

A few years ago, my friend comedian Dave DeLuca and I produced a comedy show in Los Angeles. From a performer's perspective, one of the things that makes comedy shows in Los Angeles a little different than in the rest of the country is that it is harder to get a good audience. The big clubs like the Comedy Store, Laugh Factory, and the Improv attract crowds, but those three clubs couldn't possibly keep all of LA's comedians busy all of the time. Therefore, there are a lot of smaller shows in restaurants, bars, coffee shops, theater spaces, and sometimes people's homes. I even know a couple of comedians who bought an old prison bus and converted it into a mobile comedy club.[43] With so many entertainment options, Angelenos have a lot of venues to choose from. Combine that with the fact that it can take over an hour to get from one part of the city to another, and it is not surprising that some of these shows are struggling to stay open. We produced our show at a popular bar on Santa Monica Boulevard, but even still we had a hard time filling the room. On those nights, we needed every butt in a seat that we could get. Producing a comedy show under those circumstances can be stressful, but that is not what this anecdote is about. On one particularly slow evening, an old friend of mine from Texas contacted me about seeing a show.

---

43 Shout out to Dusty Trice and Mike Frankovich, owners of the Stand Up Bus! www.standupbus.com.

Feeling in Control, Even When We're Not

I was looking forward to catching up, but also was really looking forward to having another butt in a seat. He never showed up.

He texted me after the show to apologize, and to make it up to me he offered to take me out to lunch the following day. We got together, and it was really good to see an old friend. He explained that the reason why he couldn't make the show was that he got caught in rush hour traffic coming from Orange County, and was concerned he would have an episode of road rage if he went out.

"Are you serious?" I asked.

"Yes, it has been really bad. I've been seeing someone for it" he said. Then, I asked him if he'd like to talk about it with me. He was open.

I asked him to tell me about the last time he had an episode of road rage, and he described a day when he was driving northbound on Interstate 35 through Austin. Then, he said, "All of a sudden this dude just cut me off!"

Now, I understand what people mean when they use the phrase "cut me off" but to make a point, I asked him to describe exactly what he meant by that. He said, "Okay well, I was driving in the center lane, just minding my own business, and all of a sudden this car comes out of nowhere from my right side and moves right in front of me."

"Oh, so he cut you off!" I said.

"Yeah, the dude cut me off!" he responded, not picking up on my sarcasm.

I said, "Let me ask you something, when he cut you off, did it cause you to have an accident? Did you swerve and run into another car?"

"Oh no, nothing like that," he said.

I continued, "When he cut you off, did you have to slam on your brakes or take some evasive action to avoid getting into an accident? I could see how that would be very stressful."

"Oh no, nothing like that," he said.

I continued, "When he cut you off, did this cause you to miss your exit or something? Perhaps it made you late or caused you to go out of your way."

"No, nothing like that. He just cut me off," he said.

I continued, "I just want to make sure I understand what happened. Because it sounds to me like a car changed lanes in front of you and *nothing happened*. Maybe you were momentarily inconvenienced, but nothing happened."

"No man, he cut me off!" he insisted.

Here is the thing, I know what he meant and I know how he felt in that situation. What I was trying to help him do was reframe the event. Remember that our thoughts influence how we feel and when we think of an event as "that guy cut me off," that sounds like an aggressive act. It sounds like it was intentional. Like it is a threatening act that warrants a response. However, if we think to ourselves, "That car changed lanes in front of me and nothing happened," the same situation seems a lot less likely to provoke an anger response. I explained this to him and he seemed to understand.

So then I asked, "When this guy cut you off, what did you do?"

"I got real mad," he said. Well, of course you got mad. It is called road *rage* for a reason. If the only response was an emotion, we wouldn't even be talking about it.

"What else?" I asked.

"I started tailgating him, like really close," he added. How close? "Maybe a few feet."

"Anything else?"

"I honked my horn a bunch, a lot actually," he added. "I really laid into it."

"Anything else?"

"I flipped him off a few times," he said.

"You gave him the finger? The Trudeau salute?"

"Haha, yeah."

I went on, "Okay, when you shot the bird did you do it over the dashboard/behind the windshield, or did you roll down the window and stick it outside?" Not that this matters at all, but I feel like if you are going to go through the hassle of rolling down the window to make sure that they see you, you mean business.

"Well, I was in the convertible and the top was down, so I just stuck it straight up," he said. How Californian of this Texan.

"So you are tailgating, honking, and flipping the bird. Anything else?"

"I followed him."

"You followed him? Like, to where?" I was really confused by this.

"Just for about five miles," he said.

I stopped for a moment to reflect on what my friend had just described. We all know it is dangerous to follow another car too closely, especially if you keep letting go of the steering wheel to honk the horn and throw your middle finger in the air. I summarized all of this and said to him, "Look, you endangered your *own life*, for *five miles*, because *nothing happened.*"

"Well when you put it that way it sounds kind of stupid," he said and laughed.

It *is* stupid and that is the entire point. The reaction was not a rational one made by the prefrontal cortex after weighing the pros and cons of each alternative course of action. It was a completely irrational response motivated by stress and anger, with the intention of retaliation. Retaliation for nothing happening.

My friend's behavior, although extremely unsafe, was a relatively tame reaction in comparison to some of the stories I have heard. He only followed his victim for five miles, instead of, say, all the way home. I am familiar with people who drive with "road rage kits" in the car. Basically, the kit is a bag of rocks, bricks, and other assorted items to throw at offending drivers. A colleague told me about a patient who used to pass drivers who angered him and throw nails on the road in front of their car. I wonder if those same people would throw a brick or handful of nails at someone who walked in front of them on the sidewalk—of course they wouldn't. I also have heard way more stories than I'd like to about people displaying or using firearms in traffic. And, as I shared in *The Laughing Cure*, my own father was assaulted in a road rage incident.[44] All of these incidents would fall into the category of overreacting, and the vast majority of them were probably reactions to nothing happening.

I personally believe that nothing happening is our biggest stressor. Think about all the times you have gotten stressed or angry or upset and it turned out there was no good reason for this. The

---

44 As I recall, my father was driving and angrily flipped the bird at another driver. The other driver did not seem to appreciate this because at a stoplight he got out of his car and attacked my dad.

Feeling in Control, Even When We're Not

misunderstandings, the overreactions, and all the worrying over nothing. Nothing is our most common stressor, and it is neither traffic nor bears. It is literally nothing.

I will give you another, shorter, example. This time, it involved me. I forget exactly where I was or when it happened, but I will never forget the interaction (especially if I keep sharing it). I was in a grocery store doing some shopping. Pushing my cart down each aisle as I browsed the shelves, I turned the corner into the breakfast aisle. There was a woman midway through, with her own shopping cart, examining the contents of a box of cereal. She was in the middle of the aisle, forcing me to go around her, and must not have seen me as I approached. However, she definitely noticed as I passed her and with a very indignant tone to her voice she said loudly, "Excuse me!" I asked what about and she went on, "You almost hit me, with your cart!" I didn't, but that's not the point. I answered with a smile, "So what you are saying is . . . nothing happened?" I thought to myself, *Did I hit you? No. Did you get hit? No. What do you want me to do, apologize for not hitting you? Next time I will aim better*. Literally nothing had happened, even less than in the road rage story, and she chose to get stressed.

I don't know anything about that woman, our interaction was brief and I went on with my shopping. We all have our moments, but just imagine being that sensitive to get stressed over a potential shopping cart collision. Imagine all the other encounters in life that could be stressed over. That is a lot of cumulative impact on a person's quality of life. Living in a society, we are always going to encounter other people.

When we feel rage over an incident, such as road rage, it is important to reframe our thoughts by examining the actual outcome. We need to learn to react to what *actually* happened, not what could have happened or what we thought was going to happen. When it comes to our own health and safety, there is no benefit to allowing ourselves to be affected by things that did not happen.

AND FOR THOSE WHO SKIM:

- In many cases, we become enraged over incidents where nothing serious has actually happened to us (e.g., we may have been cut off in traffic, but there was no car crash).

- Learn to react to what has happened, not what almost happened or what could have happened.

We don't all have to be able to jump out of airplanes, but at a bare minimum we should be able to handle traffic. At a bare minimum we should be able to handle shopping in public.

Learning the Hard Way
(Through an Unfortunate Series of Break-Ins)

———

I have mentioned before that I am a fairly resilient person. I don't think I could jump out of airplanes or get shot at for a living, but I tend to remain calm in most situations. Also, I would never be able to do what I do for a living if I didn't manage stress well. My speaking tour schedule can sometimes be extremely demanding, every day a new city with a new audience, and no real job security. I never know if I will be working next season or how much. As for comedy, well, I'm no Kevin Hart. It's hard to imagine putting Alyssa through college on club money. Most people could not live like we do, which is probably why most people don't. However, as much as I discuss it now, I never really had a sense that I handled stress differently than other people until I was studying psychology in graduate school. But before I get into that, let me give you some context.

I earned my undergraduate degree at the University of Texas at Austin, and right after graduating, I packed all I could into my car. I even took out the back seat to make more room for more stuff. The rest of my belongings were either sold, given away, or tossed. My plan was to start relatively fresh in New Orleans, and besides, I really didn't have much of value after years of being a broke college student. But first I had to drive to upstate New York and spend one last summer as a camp counselor. With my brother riding shotgun, in the back seat area I had the computer I bought on campus, clothes, a few small pieces of furniture, and boxes of books, tapes, and CDs (back when those things were still prized possessions). I am still amazed at how much we managed to stuff into that car. We drove the entire eighteen hundred miles in a single trip, taking turns at the wheel, with very few stops. In hindsight, I am surprised the car made the journey because shortly after arriving at the summer camp the engine caught on fire. This caused me to start graduate school in New Orleans with no car and very few possessions. Usually people have to complete grad school to be that destitute.

Graduate school itself is insanely stressful and to this day I don't recommend it to anyone.[45] Basically, it's torture that you pay for. There were thirteen of us in my beginning class, and I don't think any of us had an idea of what was in store. I remember our department chair warning us as to what we were going to experience. He said that it would be difficult and stressful, but the thing that struck me the most was when he said that from this point we were no longer consumers of knowledge, we were contributors to it. Understandably, the level of detail we were expected to know was going to be greater than in college. If we survived our first year, we would have to take an oral comprehensive exam on the field of psychology administered by our thesis committee. Mine told me to study every journal published in psychology in the last five years. Yeah, that's not stressful at all. Also, at one point our entire career depended on whether or not we could train a rat to perform a trick for one of our professors. Training a rat in a 1930s-style Skinner box[46] is hard enough, but what if your rat doesn't feel like performing on test day? I hope you have a plan B! As they say, there's always money in the banana stand.

I took it all in stride, watching my dozen peers get stressed and worry as we convened every day in a room we called the "bull pen" where a few of us had our offices. For me, this was par for the

---

45 Actually, I am referring to academic programs. I am sure more practical degrees like an MBA or Occupational Therapy, although stressful, still have their value. Also, I'm kidding.

46 Technically called an operant conditioning chamber. You may be familiar with the concept: in the chamber there is a lever that the rat can press and when it does, it receives a food pellet. After it learns to press the lever for the food pellet, then you "chain" another behavior that it must complete before it presses the lever and so on until it learns the trick. The Skinner boxes we used were not automated in any way, so we had to sit next to them with a food pellet in hand while quietly waiting for the rat to randomly touch the lever. This task alone was the source of many nightmares in graduate school.

course as I am used to being the calm one. But how I really learned I had a higher tolerance for stress than other people happened outside of school.

Unlike in Austin, where the university is in the center of the city and pretty well integrated into the culture there, the University of New Orleans was located on the edge of town. If you look at a map of New Orleans, you can see that the bulk of the city is squeezed between the Mississippi River to the south and Lake Pontchartrain to the north. Almost every cool thing in the city—the French Quarter, the Faubourg Marigny, downtown, uptown, or the Lower Garden District—is located on the river side of town. My university sat right on the lake. The area around the university was mostly residential, with big single-family homes dominating the landscape, and on-campus housing was very limited. None of my peers or the undergraduates I knew lived near campus, everyone drove in from other areas. Our class was scattered throughout the metro area. Some lived uptown, others chose to live outside the city. I chose to live in the French Quarter, because that was the area that drew me to New Orleans in the first place. I didn't move there to go to school—I applied to that school so that I could move there. Thankfully there was a bus line that ran straight from the French Quarter to the University of New Orleans Lakefront Campus down Elysian Fields Avenue, but being carless soon proved to be a major limitation, especially when trying to socialize with the other students, so I eventually bought a car.

If you've never been to New Orleans, it is an incredibly fun city. It is one of the few cities in the US with twenty-four-hour alcohol sales, and a population that knows how to party. It is the home of Cajun cuisine, voodoo, and the biggest Mardi Gras celebration this side of Panama. It is also full of beautiful architecture, such as the wrought-iron balconies and courtyards found in the French Quarter, the Creole cottages, shotgun houses, and camelback houses found throughout the city, and the antebellum mansions uptown. All of this is surrounded by gator-infested swamplands in a subtropical climate. I absolutely love New Orleans and to this day it is one of my favorite places in the world. However, it is also a city that was struggling economically well before Hurricane Katrina nearly destroyed it back in 2005. There was a lot of poverty, and pretty high crime rates. When I first moved to the French Quarter, people asked me if I was concerned about the crime.[47] Of course I wasn't. Every place has its drawbacks, and besides, I had fallen in love with the Quarter on my first visit to New Orleans and decided then that no matter what I did with my life, I had to spend at least some of it there. Despite its high crime rate, at the time I wouldn't have been happy living anywhere else.

The first time I was victimized by a crime happened a couple of weeks after I purchased the car. I came out of my apartment one morning and went to my car to find that it had been broken into. The passenger side window had been smashed and there was glass everywhere. Those CDs and tapes that I managed to haul from Austin up to New York and back down south were gone, as well as my car stereo and whatever change I happened to have in my center console. Thankfully nothing terribly important or valuable was taken from the car. I brushed the bits of broken glass aside,

---

47 Similarly, when I first moved to San Francisco, people asked if I was worried about earthquakes. Of course I wasn't. It is amusing to me that although I am not a worrier, I seem to always have people in my life who worry for me.

hopped into the driver's seat, and headed to class. In the bull pen, I told my friends what had happened and all of them seemed way more upset and concerned about it than I was. For me, the worst part of it was paying to replace my window, as my broke graduate student budget didn't include such things. I guess I was going to have to skip a few meals.

The second time I was victimized was about a week later. In almost identical circumstances, I left my apartment and walked a block down Barracks Street to find my car in a pool of broken glass and again missing the passenger side window. I was surprised because, since the first break-in, I had made it a point to keep absolutely nothing in my car. There were no tapes, no CDs, and there was an empty hole in the dashboard occupied by the space where my stereo used to be. There was nothing to be gained by breaking into my car this time. I think whoever did it did so for practice. You gotta keep your skills up, even in the smash-and-grab, car-stereo-theft game. Again, I drove to school and told my friends what had happened. They couldn't believe my car had been broken into twice in a matter of weeks. One commented, "That's why I don't go to the Quarter!" Another said, "I don't understand how you can live there!" Once again, they seemed more upset about it than I was. My major concern was paying for a new window that I hardly had the money for.

After replacing my window twice in one month, I wised up and started leaving my car unlocked. I figured that if any potential crooks happened to stumble onto my car and were tempted to see what treasures were contained within, they could just let themselves in, sparing me the need to buy yet another plate of glass. A few uneventful weeks went by and I felt like I had beat the system.

That was when I found a guy sleeping in my car. Just like any other morning, I came out to my car to drive to school. This time I found a dude sleeping in the back seat. The windows were rolled up; his head was resting on one door and his feet were pressed against the other. *At least the windows are intact*, I thought. I knocked on the glass to wake him up. "Hello," he answered. "This is my car, I need to drive it now," I told him. He apologized, gathered his things, and promptly got out of the vehicle. I didn't ask, but he explained that he had been partying hard on Bourbon Street, had a little too much, and just needed a safe place to pass out. No harm, no foul. Again, I drove to school and told my friends. "I can't believe it!" one said. "How are you so calm?" another asked. "I would be so freaked out if it was me," said another. To me, it was no big deal. There was no property damage, no window to replace, and nothing stolen. In fact, having a guy sleep in my car all night might have deterred other people from breaking in.

Then again maybe not. The very first time I went to New Orleans was for the weekend before Mardi Gras during my last year of college in Austin. It is an eight-hour drive between the two cities and I drove after class on Friday, partied all day Saturday, and drove home on Sunday. I didn't have money to spring for a hotel room, so I planned to park in a garage and retreat to the car when I got tired, which I did after the festivities of Saturday night. Early Sunday morning, I was woken up by a police officer knocking the butt of his flashlight against my window. I assumed I was in some sort of trouble. "Have you been sleeping here all night?" he asked. Yes, from maybe about three or four. "Did you see or hear anything?" at this point I noticed the purpose of his questioning. At some time during the night, the car next to me had been broken into and robbed, and I completely slept through the entire thing. That memory still makes me laugh.

Waking up and finding a stranger sleeping in your car seems like one of those events that only happens to somebody once. Yeah, not this guy. About a month or so later, it happened again. Once again, I came out of my apartment all ready and eager to go to stressful graduate school and train some rats or something. Once again, I saw the familiar image of a lone dude using my car to catch some Zs. This time he was up front, sleeping in the passenger seat. I knocked on the window. He didn't answer. I knocked a little louder. He didn't answer. Great, the last thing I need is to start my day dealing with a dead guy in my car. I opened the door, checked his breathing. He was alive, just passed out cold. So cold that he wouldn't respond to anything, not even being nudged or tapped on the cheek.

I couldn't just leave him on the sidewalk, so that was the morning that I drove to school with a passed-out stranger riding shotgun. He slept the entire drive. I arrived at campus, found a parking spot, and left him there while I went to class. I told my friends about it and they were stunned in disbelief. At the end of the day I returned to the parking lot and he was gone. I wish I could have been there when he woke up, finding himself disoriented in a strange environment on the other side of the city. If he was from out of town, I hope he was able to get home okay.

The thing is, each time I had one of these encounters it didn't seem to affect me as much as it did my friends, based on their reactions. They worried, expressed concern, and even commented that these events made them feel even more fearful than they did before. Other than the inconveniences and having to pay for window replacements, each time I laughed it off. In fact, I still laugh when I recall these events. It's hilarious. Coincidentally, around the time this was happening, we were studying stress in great detail and as I compared my reactions to those of my classmates, I began to realize that I have an unusually high tolerance for stress. I experience plenty of stress, just maybe not as much as the average person. As my brother would later point out, I "tapped into how to manage stress" at an early age and now I was starting to understand that.

I don't know how I developed my resilience. If I did, I would totally write a book, but I have some hypotheses. It probably had a lot to do with how I was raised, but unfortunately, I wasn't taking detailed notes. I wasn't a psychologist back then, I was just . . . being raised.

4

<hr>

Interview with a Real American Badass

I grew up in a military family. I owe everything I have to the United States Air Force; without it I would have never had the opportunities I was given. I have lived in other countries and all over the United States. As a child, I had great healthcare and dental work, a safe place to grow up with lots of friends, and an overall damn fine quality of life. Thanks to the military, I was prepared for and motivated to go to college and ultimately get my doctorate. All the while my father was able to support a family of four and gain marketable skills and an education. I have been around the military most of my life, and have tremendous respect for the men and women that serve in the armed forces. As an American, I fully appreciate their decision to dedicate a portion of their lives to defending us at home and abroad. Thanks to everyone who has served, especially my own father, my uncles, and their father before them, I get to tell jokes and write books for a living. This is something that I will never take for granted.

Unless Alyssa chooses to enlist, my family's involvement in the armed forces has ended with my generation. Growing up, my brother and I were a bit too rebellious to consider military service. Laziness probably factored into both of our decisions, but ultimately, it was my sense that I didn't want *potentially being shot at* to be a part of my job description that kept me out of the armed forces. My level of badassery has its limits.

I often talk about members of the military as an example of people with a high tolerance for stress, as I imagine they would need to be exceptionally resilient to handle the job. Whenever I do, the image in my mind's eye is a cross between Rambo, Nick Fury, and Chuck Norris. The kind of guy who can take on any challenge, whether it is jumping out of an airplane into waters infested with laser-headed sharks to sneak up on an enemy, or roundhouse kicking a bunch of ninjas into submission on his way to a wedding and still showing up looking dapper as hell.

Realizing that I may have read too many comic books when I was a kid, I thought it would be helpful to talk with a real-life badass. Retired Staff Sergeant Carlos "Cuban" Balestena, formerly of the 2nd Battalion, 319th Field Artillery Regiment, and 82nd Airborne Division, is one such real-life badass.

Cuban was a high school friend of Sarah's in southern Florida who served our country for seventeen years, two months, and eleven days, with his last duty station being Fort Bragg, North Carolina. Retired now, and with a daughter just a little older than Alyssa, he took time out of his day to speak with me.

BK: Can you give me a little more detail on your military career?

Cuban: Sure thing. My name is Carlos Balestena but I am known as "Cuban" by all of my Army buds. I joined the Army in July of 2001. September 11, 2001 was actually about three days away from my basic training graduation, so that was a surprise for me. From basic training I went on to take my training, my AIT,[48] in becoming a wheeled vehicle mechanic. After going through school to be a wheeled vehicle mechanic, it was January through February of 2002 that I went to Airborne School. [After] the three weeks of Airborne School, I immediately got stationed at Fort Bragg, North Carolina, home of the Airborne, and home of the Special Operations Forces.

BK: As a member of Airborne, how many jumps did you have over your career?

Cuban: Well, what was counted on paper was 108 jumps, which is actually a very . . . an extremely high feat. A very small percentage of Airborne personnel, even those who retire from the Army as Airborne, reach that. When you're a jumpmaster—I was also a jumpmaster since 2008—you get a status of being considered a "centurion jumpmaster." It [doesn't give] any more pay or an award or anything, but it's a name on a plaque, and it means a lot. [It means that] as an Airborne paratrooper, and as a jumpmaster, you were able to reach a minimum of one hundred jumps.

BK: So you were a jumpmaster for about ten years. Does that mean that you trained other paratroopers?

Cuban: Well, a jumpmaster is simply the safety guy that is

---

48 Advanced Individual Training

trained, and it's very rigorous training, very high attention to detail training, so that you can inspect the jumpers' equipment and the rigs that they are wearing, then be able to safely identify what drop zone we are supposed to be on, and then safely exit paratroopers from the aircraft. We're the first face they see when they board and the last face they see before they exit that aircraft.

BK: That's an added level of responsibility . . .

Cuban: Absolutely. Actually, an even smaller percentage of paratroopers ever even strive to become a jumpmaster.

BK: Were any of those 108 jumps into combat situations?

Cuban: None of them were into combat. I consider myself very blessed that they weren't for combat, but every Airborne operation I was ever on, minus holiday jumps with foreign jumpers, all of them were combat training. They always trained us to be ready for combat.

BK: When you first enlisted, you had specific intentions of joining Airborne, is that correct?

Cuban: Oh, yeah. Yeah, I did. My best friend growing up, his father was Special Forces, and he was an Airborne paratrooper on Fort Bragg, with the Seventh Special Forces group. He used to show us some of his old VHS videos of him and his Special Forces buddies jumping out of an aircraft over Fort Bragg, or into water. He actually did have a combat jump into Panama, I believe it was, and I thought that was really cool. I knew I wanted to join the Army, but I knew if I actually did go through with joining the Army, no matter what, I was going to be a paratrooper. I had that put in my contract when I was signing up for the Army.

BK: That was your one requirement? That you wanted to make sure that you had signed up for this Airborne training?

Cuban: Absolutely, and it came with a three thousand dollar signing bonus, so that was nice.

BK: That is interesting that you would join the Army with the stipulation that you could jump out of airplanes. Prior to joining the military, were you always attracted to extreme sports or adrenaline-junkie types of activities?

Cuban: I really wasn't. I was a Boy Scout, so camping was fun and whatnot. But as for that extreme stuff, when I enlisted, I had never even gone on an amusement park ride. Not anything major anyway. I can't really say that I really was ever much of an adrenaline junkie.

BK: So no base jumping or bungee jumping or anything like that?

Cuban: No, none of the above. Florida is rather flat, so there are not many opportunities anyhow.

BK: So what was it besides seeing those videos that was so enticing about becoming a member of Airborne?

Cuban: Well, of course, he told us all the stories of also becoming Special Forces, which is the elite of the elite, but . . . it's just the thrill. I mean, you are not in the air very long. You're falling twenty feet per second under this big, ugly round parachute that you don't steer, and there are a lot of injuries, but it's just the thought of being able to jump out of an aircraft. You get paid to jump out of an aircraft, what people normally pay a lot of money to do in free fall. And to be in an Airborne unit, where we wear a maroon beret and we wear black highly shined jump boots with our dress uniform, whereas everybody else wears what is called "low quarters"—they are just very shiny pleather shoes—it is the most elite, under being Special Forces, that you can possibly get in the United States Army.

BK: So you did it for the sweet uniform! Was it just the potential for glory and status?

Cuban: Not entirely so, but yes, that definitely did play a part in being really solidly hell-bent and set on becoming a paratrooper.

BK: Okay, now I'd like to know a little bit about the mind-set of jumping out of an airplane, and specifically what it was like the first time that you jumped. Were you anxious, nervous, stressed? Give me an idea of what was going through your mind when you first jumped out of an airplane.

Cuban: Well, to start off, it is three weeks of training in Airborne School. First, you are put through this very rigorous training. The physical training (PT) test is very, very rigorous. You also have to run everywhere you go; dining facility, barracks, training locations. The three training weeks are ground week, tower week, and then actual jump week. The first two weeks lead up to that final week of jumping out of an airplane five times before you're considered fully Airborne qualified, what we call a "five-jump chump."

During the ground week, you're just sliding around on the ground learning how to release yourself out of being dragged by a parachute, hanging in a suspended harness learning how to control your parachute and equipment, what we called "suspended agony," and jumping from twenty-four-inch platforms practicing how your body must be when you hit the ground. Then toward the end of that week, leading into the second week, you are now jumping from a thirty-four-foot platform and all you are is tethered to a rope that's held by your instructor down on the ground. You basically free-fall thirty-two feet to get the sense of what that's going to feel like, hitting the ground at sixteen to twenty feet per second. Then you got your tower week, which is more of that and jumping from a 250-foot tower, which was originally built for the 1939–1940 World's Fair in New York, and then used as an amusement park ride for civilians. Fort Benning has most of those remaining original towers. You would think it's not that big a deal but it is pretty spooky.

All of that leads us up to the morning of our first jump. We wake up at "oh-dark-thirty" is what we call it [or zero-dark-thirty, the time between 1:00 and 5:00 a.m.]. I don't even remember what time it was, but you know the sun is not coming up for hours, and you have to get into your uniform. You have got to bring your gear with you, which is your combat equipment and helmet. That usually weighs a minimum of thirty-five additional pounds, and you've got to run from the barracks all the way down to what we call the "PAX shed," or personnel shed, at the flight line.

Now you've got to get into your harness, and you're very rushed for it. The black hats (we call the instructors that because they wear a black ball cap) are yelling, "Let's go. Let's get in your rig." If you are taking too long, they are really yelling at you. They try to keep it fairly low stress, but you can tell they are building you up for it. You are sitting there for hours waiting on the aircraft, or even when the aircraft arrives, waiting on your turn. Now, you're just running through your mind, *Oh man, am I forgetting anything?* Or, *I gotta keep my eyes open, chin in chest, feet and knees together, the knees locked to the rear, body bent slightly forward at the waist, so that the parachute* . . . I could talk the full gambit, it is all just going through your mind, *Okay, I don't want to forget this. I don't want to forget this.*

Finally, you are being led onto the aircraft: a small, dark, and cramped aircraft. It's hot in there. You're starting to get really, really nervous. You're flying around for twenty to thirty minutes, then all of a sudden the doors open up. There are small, little doors on either side of the aircraft. The wind, cool wind, blows in, and the nerves pick up a little bit, but it is very weird, an unexplainable nerve, that it's almost a calm. What I always tell everyone is the best I can say it is, I blacked out. I knew what I was doing, so I didn't truly black out, but it's as if my mind went completely into training mode, and it said, *Okay, I'm doing exactly what these guys told me to do.*

BK: It sounds to me as if you were so well trained that you put your faith in that training?

Cuban: Absolutely. I couldn't say it any better. You're putting your faith in not only that training, but that instructor, that jump-master's hand, and you're saying, *All right, he's going to take my static line out of my hands.* Our parachutes were already attached via cable to the aircraft, so it pulls our parachute out for us. We're not pulling our own parachute like in the civilian free-fall world. But you got to trust that, first of all, the guy in front of you does the right thing, so he doesn't trip or throw his equipment in your face or something. Then you've got to trust that the Safety in that door is going to grab that static line from you at the right moment, so that you can just concentrate on making a 90-degree turn and just jumping out of that door. "Up six and out thirty-six" is what we always say. You try to jump up six inches and out thirty-six inches.

BK: At what point in your career did the nerves go away?

Cuban: So with the first five jumps, everything is fairly mechanical. You have that nerve still with you, but even after all those years, and I hit jump number one hundred, I hit jump number 108, I was always asked, "Do you still feel nervous when you jump? Do you still feel scared?" I've never once felt scared, but I've always had an amount of nerves. I guess, I could best say a level of nerves, and I always told my soldiers, "The day that you lose those nerves is the day that it's time for you to get out of this community, to stop jumping out of [an] aircraft." The saying that we have in the Army is "stay alert, stay alive." That little twinge in the back of your neck, in the back of your mind, is what gives you that "stay alert." As long as you stay alert and you do what everyone tells you to do, to the T, to the letter, then you'll be all right.

BK: Gotcha. Before signing up with the Army and obviously before joining the Airborne Division, how would you say that you handled stress back in your civilian days?

Cuban: Well, stress was . . . I mean, those days were high school days, they were middle school days, they were elementary school days. I dealt with stress just like anybody else did. Sometimes you acted out. Sometimes you cried. Sometimes you were scared and just completely immobilized. It was just the general growing up nerves and growing up fears, and I handled it just like anybody else. I didn't have any better coping mechanisms than anybody else. I mean, I was able to differentiate between what's a true worry and then what's, ah, well, you know, *I'll be worried about this, but I'll live through it.*

BK: It sounds like your coping mechanisms were on par with other people. What about after serving in Airborne and the Army?

Cuban: If I could jump out of what some call a "perfectly good aircraft" (they've never flown in an Air Force aircraft) at a thousand feet above the ground, with a parachute packed by some eighteen-year-old that had only sixteen weeks of Army training to learn to be a parachute rigger, not a college graduate but just another fellow paratrooper, and just keep my eyes open, my chin in my chest, and just jump—put my knees to the breeze—I can really deal with about anything.

BK: That's perfect. That's the quote I want to use right there. What I've been telling people is if I can jump out of an airplane, traffic is no big deal.

Cuban: No kidding. Forget it. Traffic, come on.

BK: In your day-to-day life now in retirement, do things bother you? Does it give you a perspective on life? How does it influence your living now?

Cuban: The same things that bothered you, that bother anybody else, are the same things that bother me, but I think I'm more able than most people to just sit back and say, *You know what? It could be worse. I'm alive.* Again, if I can jump out of all that, if I could just put my knees to the breeze and just let it rip, really, what the hell else is going to really bother me? What do I got to worry about?

BK: One last question: you and I both have little girls. Which do you think is more stressful, serving in the Army or raising a daughter?

Cuban: Ha ha! I have to say the daughter! In the Army,

I usually had a minimum of ten to forty "children" that I was responsible for. I was responsible for their health, their welfare, and the accomplishment of our mission. I've taken them to war and returned with 100 percent. But having Lola Rose? One little girl stopped my whole life! Now I have this fragile (but furious) little girl and all I ever think about is, is she safe, and am I doing everything I can and right by her?

BK: There you go, I guess I am an American badass after all. Thanks, Cuban!

5

The Choices
We Make

As much as I talk about being highly resilient myself, I have to admit that I am not Superman. Things get to me. Usually, I only get stressed about the bears in my life, like when the kitchen of my Montreal condo was suddenly turned into a direct access point to the earth. But there are occasions when I will let minor, stupid things get the best of me. As you know, my favorite example of something trivial to stress about is traffic. Generally, I don't get too worked up in traffic. To me, traffic is just cars moving slow. Cars are *safer* when they are moving slow! *So what* if you get in an accident going ten miles an hour on Interstate 70? What kind of damage could that possibly cause? Not much, I imagine, as I answer my own hypothetical question. Still, I do set my GPS to avoid traffic whenever I can.

In the interest of full disclosure, I will tell you about a recent experience when I got *super* stressed in traffic. I forget where it happened, but it certainly wasn't in Colorado as it is way too difficult to let anything stress you out in this state. I was doing one of my seminars, at some hotel somewhere. Generally, my speaking gigs are in hotel conference centers and usually, to make things easy on myself, I spend the night in the hotel that I will be speaking in. I find that it makes for a really easy commute. My morning goes like this: I roll out of bed, throw on some clothes, and take the elevator downstairs. Well, this time when my agent went to make my travel arrangements, we found out that the hotel had sold out on the night I needed. No big deal, I would just take whatever was nearby and have a slightly longer commute in the morning. There must have been a big event (even bigger than my own!) going on at that time because my travel agent ended up booking me a room about eight miles away. Still, this is no big deal. I'm no diva; I don't mind driving.

The problem was that when I arrived at the hotel, the clerks greeted me and asked if I was there for the "event." I mistakenly thought they were referring to my speaking engagement and said yes. So now it is in my head that I am going to be speaking there in the morning. I went to bed unconcerned, expecting everything to go as usual. When I woke up, I leisurely took my time getting ready before taking the elevator downstairs. I met someone in the lobby and asked for directions to the conference center. They didn't have one. This wasn't the first time this had happened, so I realized pretty quick that I was at the wrong place. What made this morning different is that I went to sleep completely convinced that I was in the right spot for the talk and made no effort to double-check just to be sure. I was now standing in the lobby of the wrong hotel and had no idea where I was supposed to be.

I was in another time zone from my agency, so I wasn't able to contact anyone to quickly remedy the situation. I actually had to get on a computer and look for the brochure online to get the address. It was eight miles away, the GPS said it would take about fifteen minutes to get there, and I had thirty until I was supposed to start. It was going to be tight, but things were still under control.

I arranged for the hotel to hold my luggage, hopped in the car, and hit the road. A few blocks later, I took the on-ramp onto the interstate and found myself in some very dense, slow-moving traffic. My GPS updated my estimated time of arrival, showing that the trip was now expected to take over twenty-five minutes. I was going to be late, and I got seriously anxious. I felt my heart rate increase, I became agitated, and I started to perspire and worry. I thought about the two hundred or so people I was going to inconvenience by showing up late. I worried about my reputation, and I worried about how I would be perceived. Ironically, I was on my way to a seminar about stress management where I was planning on discussing traffic and worry. So yeah, it happens to all of us.

However, when I realized I was beginning to succumb to my stress response I started to direct the activity of my prefrontal cortex into a more productive area, and to think about something else, as I have suggested we should do in these situations. I interrupted my flow of worry and reminded myself that the situation was out of my control. *There is nothing I can do about this traffic. Sometimes people are late. Being late happens. It is not the end of the world.* Suddenly I started to calm down. Ultimately, I started the seminar about five minutes late. Were those five minutes worth suppressing my immune system or enduring any of the other physical effects of stress? Of course not. Even if I was five hours late, the pain and suffering that stress wreaks on the body would not be worth it. People are late all the time—people even regularly have to cancel engagements. It is unfortunate and inconvenient, but certainly not a bear.

Getting to the Gym Across the Street

The thing about writing a book is that sometimes you hit your stride, cranking out pages and pages of engaging text, and sometimes . . . well, sometimes you can't even force it. While pounding out pages isn't necessarily hard physical labor, writing can be terribly frustrating and terribly stressful, especially when you are working on a deadline. Here I am, writing this on a Sunday evening. All weekend long, I have known what I want to write but I have been having a hard time getting it out.

To help clear my head, I put my computer away and asked Sarah to get Alyssa ready to go for a drive. Although it is early November in Colorado, we've been enjoying moderate temperatures for the past few weeks, which we have been taking advantage of at the nearby parks and zoo (and still no bear attacks!). Getting out into the world did the trick. As soon as I got out of the house, the ideas for how to start this section started flowing. Some of them were better than others, of course. By the time this gets into your hands, I hope I chose well.

I didn't have to let you in on that thought process, but I did so because it serves as a good example of something I mentioned earlier that you may have forgotten: if you don't like the way you feel, change your thoughts. This is probably one of the best pieces of advice I can share, so it is worth returning to. I felt frustrated and maybe even a little stressed so I took steps to change my thoughts. Sometimes a change in environment or activity is precisely what we need to kick-start different activity in our prefrontal cortex. For whatever reason, I had hit a major roadblock in my writing process. A "writer's block" if you will. I'm pretty sure I just made up a new term there—you can use it if you like.

In the previous sections I have hopefully made the point that feeling in control is key to remaining calm and reducing the overall impact of stress in our lives. If I haven't, maybe you shouldn't have been skimming after all. And you wonder why you got that "D" in history. I feel you—I wasn't a very good student either. Okay, here is your recap: being resilient means having the right kind of activity in the prefrontal cortex so that your amygdala doesn't react to everything in our world as a potential danger. In other words, being resilient means having the right kinds of thoughts in your head, and those thoughts relate to how well you feel you can handle whatever situation you are facing. I am sure you have heard the phrase "power of positive thinking" or something like that being spewed by so-called motivational gurus, but there really is a kernel of truth to phrases like that.[49]

Maybe you don't have those positive thoughts. Instead, maybe you have a tendency to worry. Maybe you are quick to anger or maybe you tend to focus on negativity. I find that some people aren't even aware of how negative they really are. Here's an example: as I mentioned it is November, and so far on my Facebook feed, I have seen at least nine people post complaints about early Christmas decorations or music. Why? Because Thanksgiving is the next holiday on the calendar? So what, are cities supposed to hang turkey lights for the few weeks after Halloween? Decorations and lights make people happy, particularly now that daylight savings is upon us and people are leaving work in darkness. It is a complaint I hear every year, at least a few times a year, and it is just unnecessary negativity. Just watch, in a couple of months these same people will be complaining that the decorations are still up.

Or, perhaps you would just like to learn how to become more resilient. Because, let's face it, we can all probably benefit from managing stress better.

The good news is we have a lot of potential to change our thought patterns, our reactions, our impulsive behaviors, and even our worrying. As I mentioned previously, our brain has a characteristic called neuroplasticity which gives us the ability to learn

---

49 I've never read it, but Norman Vincent Peale's book *The Power of Positive Thinking* (New York, NY: Prentice Hall, 1952) has influenced generations of thinkers and hacks alike.

new things. The bad news is that it ain't easy. It takes effort, and in some cases, it takes a whole lot of effort. If real, lasting change was truly easy to accomplish, way fewer people would suffer from hypertension, diabetes, erectile dysfunction, or any stress-related physical condition. If change was easy, there would be way fewer people suffering from anxiety disorders or depression. If change was easy, I don't think road rage would be an issue and I certainly would not have that great story to share with you. If change was easy, there would be no need for a book like this and I would definitely be writing about something else.

One of the reasons that change is so difficult for us is that throughout our lives we have practiced behaviors that were gratifying, rewarding, or easy. Our brains have become accustomed to using them. Back when I used to report to an office for work, I would come home between five and six o'clock. Once home, my brain had a multitude of behavioral options to choose from. I could change into my exercise clothes and go to the gym across the street (the activity I consciously wanted to do). I could go for a vigorous walk around the neighborhood (an alternate). I could practice my Spanish or read a book or even learn something new (another alternate). I could also plop down on the couch and flip through the channels on TV for a few hours. Guess which option my brain chose most often? If you guessed hit the gym, I appreciate your optimism but I have to admit that the couch won that battle almost every time. It was a slaughter, really. The gym never had a chance. In my defense it was never a conscious choice made by my prefrontal cortex, but rather something my brain did automatically or out of habit. After the decision had been made by my brain, I could rationalize it, thinking to myself, *I'll just decompress for a bit before hitting the gym*, but deep down I knew what was going to happen. Sitting on the couch was the easiest option, and if I was sufficiently entertained it was also the most rewarding. In comparison, going to the gym required so much additional effort, and was probably going to hurt.

I am sure that many of you may be losing a similar battle day after day. Oh, not you? Right, it must be all the people who aren't reading this book that are contributing to the obesity epidemic. My readers are all health nuts, no wonder you didn't relate to my chocolate example. Exercise may not be difficult but it requires way more effort than sitting on our ass. There are people out there who have exercised so much throughout their lives that their brain has become accustomed to that activity, and they continue to do so, again out of habit. Unfortunately, these people are in the minority, but regardless I am sure you can understand the example so far.

Now, there have been moments in my life where I have been filled with motivation to exercise more and get healthier. Against the judgment of my brain, I would force myself to go to that gym. I would force myself to get that exercise each day. In the past when I have done this, I will admit that every day was slightly easier than the day before it, but it still required a great deal of effort to resist the call of that sweet, sweet couch. And every time, after a brief period of regularly working out, I reverted back to my old habit. I think most people will be able to relate to this.

Change is hard, but not impossible. For example, despite the five-year age difference, my brother, Jon, and I had very similar habits growing up. Neither of us were into sports or terribly physically active. Actually, that's a nice way to put it. The truth is we were lazy, very lazy. Super lazy. We even invented a dance that we could do while lying on our backs on the couch. And we were so lazy that we only did the couch dance to one song when it played on MTV, "Unbelievable" by EMF. (You gotta admit that was a great song—they even sampled Andrew Dice Clay. That song came out in 1990, and I haven't done the dance since, so don't ask.) One dance? While lying down? *That's* lazy.

Given our similar proclivities toward sloth, you may be surprised to learn that about twenty years ago Jon started exercising on a regular basis and has yet to stop. In fact, he has been active so long that I believe it has become his habit. He gets anxious when he doesn't have an opportunity to exert energy. While he changes the activity—from volleyball to CrossFit, rock climbing to Krav Maga—he has remained consistently active the entire time. When he comes home from work, his brain is excited about hitting the gym or the volleyball court or whatever. He still has the potential to get lazy, but for all practical purposes he has successfully changed his behavior.

(By now you might be wondering if my drive to overcome writer's block took me past Christmas decorations and a gym. Umm . . . maybe.)

The laziness I have just described is not related to our stress response, but hopefully you can see the analogy. Imagine that you have spent your entire life practicing a particular set of behaviors. If you are quick to anger, sorrow, or worry, it means that for some reason your brain finds that behavior to be more gratifying, or rewarding, or easier to perform than remaining calm. Let's say every time you felt threatened or out of control you exploded with an outburst of anger. Now, when you find yourself driving in traffic you experience rage and automatically lash out at other drivers. Should you decide to change that behavior, and you can, it is going to require effort. When you enter that triggering situation, you are going to have to consciously choose to engage alternative responses. Maybe you engage a calming exercise like breathing or counting, or maybe you just turn on the radio, anything to help redirect your thoughts. Who knows why you react this way— maybe you picked up the behavior after a lifetime of experiences or maybe it was triggered by a single event. Actually, it probably doesn't matter why you react that way, only that you start actively choosing another reaction. In the same way, it didn't matter why my ass liked being parked on the couch, only that I started walking it across the street to the gym.

It might sound simple, but it is tough, and it is tough to remember to redirect your thoughts day after day after day. A lot of people attempt to make changes like that, and most of them relapse into their previous response, but remember that if Jon can teach his brain to love exercise then you can probably learn to not get so pissed at traffic.

I'll take the gym analogy even further. If you have been regularly exercising your entire life, you may not relate, but I am betting most of my readers aren't gym rats. The thing about exercise is that it is work; exercise is strenuous physical activity and the longer we go without it, the harder it is for us to carry it out. Ironic, because we start our lives with quite a bit of exercise, only we call it "play" throughout childhood. Some of us will continue this pattern into our teenage years and segue into sports, but others such as yours truly, will find other interests that involve far less physical exercise (if only reading comic books was an aerobic activity). As we head further into adulthood, far too many of us enter into very sedentary lifestyles where we sit at work for about a third of our day, sit in traffic, and then sit on the couch to decompress after all that sitting. Our bodies adapt to this lack of activity and we become flabby and our muscles atrophy. More Rocky Road, less Rocky Balboa. Given our condition after years of disuse, it is no wonder our brain thinks it is much easier and more gratifying to do nothing. When we finally decide to make a change in our life, don our finest spandex, and hit the local gym, the experience can be difficult and likely not as immediately rewarding as we fantasized. However, if we somehow manage to drag ourselves back for another round the next day, working out becomes less of a drag. As we continue to force ourselves, it becomes increasingly easier and maybe even enjoyable. We all know this; and yet, we continue to sit on the couch. Becoming resilient requires the same kind of persistence. If we've somehow lived life without developing good stress-management skills, when we decide to do something about it, we are going to find it difficult and awkward. However, over time it will become more comfortable.

The brain is not a muscle; it does not grow bigger with repeated usage. Regardless of how hard you try, no amount of mental activity is going to make a part of your brain push a bump out of the skull.[50] Muscles, on the other hand, can get massive with use. The brain does not get bigger, but as I mentioned previously, it

---

50 Contrary to what the phrenologists believed.

can modify itself and rearrange things in response to usage. Some areas get more complex by adding new connections between cells, whereas areas that are used less often are reduced to compensate. Sarah's brain has recently learned to play the piano. We don't travel with our own MRI machine, but I would imagine that the part of her brain involved in that activity has grown from "nonexistent" to "a little more complex." Everything in the brain works this way; through repeated practice of a behavior, we develop the area associated with that behavior. Similarly, the more we practice resilient thinking, the more we develop the left side of our prefrontal cortex.

So how do we get there? It's much easier to list the steps on how to get to the gym across the street, that's why the analogy works, but now we have to get practical. Some of the things I have discussed so far are worth repeating, because all of them will help exercise that prefrontal cortex. Here they are then, in a skimmer-friendly format.

IN ORDER TO CHANGE OUR BEHAVIOR, WE NEED TO:

- Learn to assess our stressful situations to determine if they are actually threatening and if there is something we can do about them.

- Learn to redirect our brain away from worrisome or negative thoughts. If simply changing our thoughts doesn't work, then we can change our environment or activity.

- Repeatedly practice the behavior we want to exhibit.

6

Three Days in Xpujil (Jon's Story)

I have mentioned that I think that all stressful events could be viewed as situations where the brain does not perceive that it has any control. Bear attacks, traffic jams, unanticipated home repairs, people passing us in the grocery store, jumping out of airplanes, car break-ins, and being late for important events are all situations that we may or may not have some control over, but we can feel as if we do. How? Well, we can read up on bears before we go hiking, contract trustworthy real estate managers to look over our property, or sign up for a three-week-long paratrooper training course. In other words, we can take the necessary steps to prepare for situations we may likely encounter.

However, we cannot possibly anticipate every difficult situation that we may find ourselves in. This is where our ability to solve problems comes in handy. Our prefrontal cortex, perhaps as part of providing us with our resilience, is the area of the brain we use to solve problems. Another way to think about stressful events from the perspective of your brain is that they represent problems that need to be solved. Threatening problems, sure, but problems nonetheless. Therefore, if we have well-developed problem-solving skills, we are more likely to respond to a stressful event with the confidence that we can influence the outcome. In other words, we will respond as if we feel some level of control.

I have mentioned my brother a few times so far throughout this book. He was very kind in saying that I was "unaffected by stress" from an early age. That is an exaggeration of course, as I have given you several examples of when I have been affected by stress, but kind. I do seem to have a higher tolerance for stress than average, but so does he. Having the same parents (at least that is what they tell us), my brother, Jon, and I share 50 percent of our genes. We were also raised together, so naturally you would expect there to be some similarities between us. Like me, Jon is very resilient and skilled at problem-solving.

After he graduated college, Jon took an awesome job as an adventure tour guide for a company based in Northern California.[51] He drove a fifteen-passenger van full of mostly European tourists to sites all across the United States and he did so in the age before cell phones and GPS, and without access to the internet. As I use my smartphone to make all of my travel plans, navigate cities, and keep up with my work, it is amazing

---

51 While working on my doctorate, I spent a summer working for the same company but I did way fewer tour routes. I had one group of Italian tourists who, via their translator, asked me what I did when I wasn't leading tours. I told them I was studying psychology and, funnily enough, three of them happened to be psychologists.

to think back on how we managed those things just a couple of decades ago. Jon was so good at his job that the company eventually trusted him to lead tours south of the border into Mexico (the Spanish he picked up living in Texas helped too). Once tour leaders crossed the border, they were practically cut off from the home office in California, so only those with a demonstrated ability to think on their feet were given those assignments. You can imagine that my brother had a hell of a time working on that job, and has some great stories. I thought one of his encounters in particular was such a good story that I urged him to write it.[52] He has given me permission to share it here.

> One day while driving from Palenque to Tulum, a trip that would normally take about ten hours, the van broke down. I had a van full of tourists in the middle of nowhere along the Guatemalan border and the van simply stopped running. I pulled over and tried to crank the engine and got nothing. I couldn't see any obvious problems with the engine; whatever had gone wrong was beyond my ability to repair. I had to assess the situation. There we were, broken down alongside a single lane road with no shoulders in the middle of the southern Mexican jungle. There was no traffic on the road and no sign of civilization. I hadn't seen a town for miles.
>
> Of course, my tourists were concerned, so I had to react quickly and with confidence. I took whatever food and water we were carrying down from the roof in case we had to wait for an extended amount of time. I told them that everything

---

52 He originally wrote this story for his book *Seven Months Deep*, published in 2004. The version presented here has been edited slightly.

was cool and that I was going to figure it out. After all, "It's an adventure tour."

About fifteen minutes later an El Camino came down the road heading in the same direction that we were traveling. I stood in the middle of the road and flagged them down. I asked them how far it was to the nearest town and what it had to offer. Xpujil was the nearest town, they told me. It was a half hour away, although it didn't have anything: no hotels, no gas station, and no traveler amenities at all. They told me that the nearest town past Xpujil was Chetumal, about an additional three hours away on the Belizean border. Chetumal did have a gas station and a few hotels.

I caught a ride with them to Xpujil. I told the tourists just to sit tight in the van and eat and drink and I would be back as soon as possible.

I hopped into the back of the El Camino and rode for thirty minutes until we arrived at Xpujil. It was a tiny, dusty town and I was dropped off right in the center of it. Looking around, I guessed the town had less than five hundred inhabitants. There was a small restaurant, which also doubled as a grocery store. There was an open-faced concrete building with yellow paint spelling out the word "*Taller*" and across the street there was a similar open-faced building with the word "Autobus" written on it. In the median of the two sides of the roads were a few parked taxis.

Everybody in town stared at me as I went over to the mechanics and asked them to look at the van thirty minutes down the road. I hired a taxi for the mechanics and two minivan taxis to pick up my thirteen stranded tourists. When we returned to the van, the mechanics looked under the hood and then under the van and told me, "*Esta chingada*"— the van was fucked. It would require attention in their shop for three days.

Three days! I asked why it would be so long. They told me that it was probably the major disk that broke, and that they would have to go to Chetumal and purchase the piece before they could install it. The installation would take an afternoon.

I got all of the tourists' belongings from the top of the van, loaded them and myself into the minivan taxis, and headed back to Xpujil. We were dropped off at the restaurant and I told them to hang out while I figured out what to do. *What do I do with thirteen tourists that don't speak a lick of Spanish*, I thought. The tour was to end in a few days in Cancun, so I thought that would be the best place for them to wait for me. They could stay in a hotel and get by speaking English; besides, it is beautiful and there are a ton of things to do. I walked over to the Autobus building and asked when the next bus for Cancun was due.

"Tomorrow," the young girl told me.

These people could not stay the night in this town. There weren't even hotels and we would have to pitch tents on the side of a dirt road. I went to the taxi stand and asked what they would charge for a trip to Cancun. It would be a twelve-hour trip for the taxi drivers and they would have to take three minivans. I tried to bargain with them, but they knew I was desperate. The total came to four hundred dollars and the nearest cash machine was in Chetumal, so I had to borrow the money from the tourists. I gave all of them the name and number of the hotel they were to go to and told them that I would call to make sure they were all right. I wrote the same information down for the taxi drivers. With a borrowed four hundred dollars, they were on their way to Cancun.

Next, the mechanics and I had to organize a way to transport the broken-down fifteen-passenger van to their shop. We took two minivans back down the road and brought some short chains. We attached a chain from the front of my van to one of theirs. The return trip took an hour because of the weight dragging on the minivan. By the time we returned, it was dark out, but they understood my time pressure and began to take the van apart. Because I had absolutely nothing else to do, I watched them as they worked. I had dinner at the local restaurant and grocery store; in fact, I had every single meal for the next three days at that place. Luckily the restaurant had a television so I was able to pass a good amount of the time watching horrible Mexican programming. As there was no hotel, when the mechanics finished, I grabbed a blanket and spread out on a bench seat inside my van and prepared for bed. I asked them about the next steps and they said that we would definitely have to go to Chetumal for the part.

I awoke the next day to the sound of the mechanics working on my van. They had disassembled the entire thing. They jacked it up on a couple of cinder blocks on the dirt road in front of the shop. From the looks of the operation it seemed a bit ad hoc, but from some of my other experiences in Mexico, and from what these guys were explaining to me, they knew their work. When the van was opened up it seemed like a human body having heart surgery. They were right about the problem and showed me the broken disk. The disk was supposed to be connected to the bar that spun the back tires and propelled the vehicle. This disk was broke as a joke, definitely *chingada*.

There were two mechanics: the owner of the shop, who was an older man with a great sense of humor and a hard work ethic, and a younger man who had moved there only a couple of years prior after completing his mechanic training in the large, northern city of Monterrey. He was exceptionally bright and knew a lot about auto mechanics, and was an equally hard worker. These two guys worked well into the first evening and began again very early the next morning.

The second day was Sunday, and in Mexico nothing is open on Sunday. Rigid Catholicism coupled with low-paying jobs has created a culture rooted in weekday siestas and chilling on Sundays. The young mechanic, who was even younger than I was, spent a good portion of the day going to junkyards in the town to see if there was an extra part that would fit the bill. There was nothing. With nothing to do, I spent that entire day at the restaurant store watching television and drinking Nescafé.

The monotony of my day was broken up by a parade of sorts that lasted for a couple of hours. I am not sure what the parade was for, but the young mechanic invited me to watch it with him. There were decorated cars and residents marching through the streets. Mexico has a very interesting religious culture. Prior to the colonial conquest of "New Spain" by Hernán Cortés, Mexicans practiced paganism. Aztecs, Mayans, and Olmecs, to name a few of the major groups of people indigenous to Mexico, practiced multi-deity religions. As history tells us, Cortés boated his Spanish ass over to Mexico, and forcefully imposed the Catholic religion. An interesting mix of paganism and Catholicism was then born where many Catholic saints took on properties of indigenous deities. The saints are recognized and celebrated on different days and because there are so many saints, religious celebrations are very common. Because Mexicans are broke, the celebrations are usually limited to decorating cars and parading down streets. I guessed that this parade had something to do with some saint or another.

Although the parade was a nice diversion, the day for me concluded just as the previous had: asleep early on a bench of the van. All I could do was wait for Monday and hope that Chetumal had the part we needed.

On the third day, the young mechanic and I went together to Chetumal. It was early, and for some reason the taxi stand was empty so we hitchhiked for the three-hour trip, bringing the huge broken disk with us. The mechanic was used to going to Chetumal and knew his way around well. We were dropped off in the center of town at one of the major auto part shops. They didn't have what we needed. We proceeded to visit every auto parts store within walking distance, only to discover that none of them had the part. We then hailed a taxi and went to every auto parts store in town, again finding nothing. "Well, so much for getting a new one," the mechanic said as he directed the taxi driver to take us to a junkyard.

We went to every junkyard in Chetumal and again turned up nothing. I was getting very nervous because without this piece I could not operate the van and I really didn't want to have to think of alternatives. Meanwhile, I had a group of international tourists who didn't speak Spanish sitting in Cancun. If I couldn't get the van repaired in Xpujil, I'd have to have it towed to Cancun, which would involve getting a tow truck from Cancun to make the twelve-hour roundtrip journey. Then, I'd have to find a mechanic there and wait for them to install the new disk. The only other alternative was to call management and have another van driven down all the way from Santa Rosa, California, a four- to five-day trip for them.

"*No te preocupes*," the mechanic told me: not to worry. He had a plan C.

He told me that he was going to solder the broken disk together, so once again we returned to the Chetumal town center, this time to buy some solder sticks at the local market. I also went to a bank machine and withdrew as much money as I could, then we had the Chetumal taxi driver drive us back to Xpujil. After passing through military checkpoints and a hundred huge-ass speed bumps along the way, we returned after dark. He and the older mechanic began the soldering. The work had to be done precisely, and minor misplacements of the parts would result in the job not being able to be done. Therefore, soldering the disk was a time-consuming process. A couple of hours went by and it was very late. I invited the mechanics to the restaurant for some Nescafé and dinner. They took me up on a beer but had to go home to their wives and children. As it turned out, the young mechanic was a husband and father of two. He seemed more grown up and more responsible than I had ever been in my entire life.

As I again slept in the van that night, I really hoped it would be my final night of uncomfortable sleep. It had been three nights and I really wanted a bed and a shower and a decent meal. Also, I was really getting concerned about my tourists, and I had to worry about the new group of Europeans who were expecting me to begin their tour from Cancun to Mexico City in the next few days.

My fourth day in Xpujil began early again. The mechanics continued soldering the disk at the crack of dawn. When I woke up, it seemed that they were about a quarter of the way finished and I thought it would be another long day. I spoke with the mechanics and, although they assured me that it would work out and not to worry, they seemed to be losing their assurance. I watched them for a while before going to the restaurant store for some Nescafé. I simply could not relax that day. I had been in the tiniest of towns sitting at a grocery store that nobody except for me patronized as a restaurant for three days so far. For variation, I walked around the town, which was nothing more than a couple of dirt roads. I walked back and forth from the mechanic shop to the restaurant every thirty minutes that morning to watch their progress. After a couple of hours, the hardworking mechanics came to me and told me that they had good news.

Anticipating that they would tell me they were finished soldering, they instead told me that they found a used disk from one of their friends and that they were going to return to the original plan. I was the most relieved I have ever been in my life, as they worked for the remainder of the afternoon replacing the part. By the late afternoon, they completed the work.

I thought about the work they had just done and the extent of my skills and knowledge, and it was this point that had a profound, lasting effect on me. There I was, a college graduate, literally helpless in this situation. I felt unskilled since I had had to depend upon the mechanical expertise of these poor Mexican guys in this dusty town. I remembered some of the books that I had read and some of the discussions I had taken part in and some of the papers that I had written. I also thought about my skill base and my former jobs of cashiering and making pizzas. I looked at these two guys who had a mechanic shop constructed out of four concrete slabs and who lived in a town with dirt roads and no gas station and I became humbled.

Those guys worked their asses off and knew enough about automobiles to correctly identify the problem. They were incredibly resourceful and were going to get the job done at any expense. They worked long hours and dedicated themselves to fixing that van, just so I could drive some Germans to see pyramids. It was at that point in my life when I became very appreciative and humble and realized that, although I had gone through a four-year college, I really didn't know anything practical. It was then that I knew I had to acquire some skills. It was then that I decided to further my education.

I thanked these two guys profusely and they asked for a fair price. I gave them double and I hopped back in the driver's seat once again.

I love that story, and I hope that you can see why. The mechanics in that small Mexican town definitely saved the day for my brother and his tourists. Jon may have felt that he was lacking in practical, mechanical skills, but he really deserves a lot of credit for his problem-solving skills. When faced with an extremely difficult situation, he quickly came up with a plan and took action. He even came up with a backup plan and a backup to his backup, just in case things didn't work out. He was patient, optimistic, and handled the situation to the best of his ability. There is no training or book that can prepare you for situations like that. Not everyone can deal with such an event that effectively, and it makes an older brother proud.

7

Puzzles, Games, and Bear Attacks

oincidentally, as I have been writing the last couple of chapters, my brother, Jon, and our parents have been visiting Sarah and me in Denver for a week. I think they are mainly here to see our daughter, but if having a child helps bring the family together, so be it. It is fortuitous having them here precisely as I enter into my discussion of how we can become more resilient through practice, because I was planning on referencing them anyway, as well as the importance of continuing that practice to maintain resilience.

Before sharing my brother's breakdown story (the van, not him), you might recall I used a muscle analogy to describe how we can "strengthen" parts of our brain and develop particular patterns of activity. Just as muscles adapt to repeated exercise, through repeated practice of a behavior, our brain becomes more adept at performing that behavior. Think about any piece of factual information you have learned. Maybe you spent your childhood memorizing sports stats, comic book characters, or psychological phenomena, whatever—to convince your brain to make the physical changes required to commit your information to memory, you had to practice. Whether purposeful or not, you repeatedly exposed yourself to the information until it became stored somewhere in the folds of your cortex. The same is true for your skills. You probably don't remember it, but you learned to walk and talk through practice. You learned to read and write by practicing—unless you can't, but then how are you doing it now? Is someone reading this to you? Is this a bootleg audiobook? You can tell me, I promise I won't get mad.

We have a natural period in our lives when our brain has an opportunity to practice and acquire an enormous amount of information and skills. We call that period "childhood." My daughter Alyssa is learning new things every day, and her brain is developing in response to her experiences. This month she has learned to turn light switches on and off (standing on a step), how water faucets work, and at nineteen months (today), I think she is pretty close to wanting her own iPad. She's also learning a few other things that she may not wish me to reveal, but one thing that makes me an especially happy daddy is that she shows a lot of interest in puzzles and other prefrontal cortex exercisers.

Having my parents handy, I interviewed them a bit and they told me that I was the same way. When I was about Alyssa's age, I had a collection of jigsaw puzzles that I enjoyed solving and was really attracted to toys that allowed me to build things, like Lincoln Logs and blocks. Because I was destined to be a total genius, I used to build roads for my toy cars out of books. Yeah, sure beats reading them. Similarly, my brother was very into Legos and would spend hours building things. One thing both my parents mentioned about my childhood was that I never seemed to let things get to me and always appeared to be fairly happy. Not that I wasn't a significant source of stress for them—my mother tells me that one day I followed a dog a few blocks down the street, causing her to majorly freak out. I bet I was an interesting child. Sarah was very hands-on and observational as a child. When she was about Alyssa's age, her mother was sewing dresses and Sarah mimicked her use of scissors. Her father was a carpenter, and she had lots of access to lumber and tools. When she was a little older, she built a tree fort in the backyard that was so big the city made her family take it down.

So, hypothetically speaking, if someone managed to make it all the way to adulthood without developing good stress-management skills, how would they obtain them? I'm, uh . . . asking for a friend. That friend is you, by the way. Well, unfortunately, there is no quick fix, no magnetic field or nutritional supplement that is going to suddenly produce an abundance of activity in the left side of our prefrontal cortex when we encounter our next stressor. If we want problem-solving skills, we just have to start, you know . . . solving problems. There simply is no substitute. If you want big muscles, you have to exercise them, and if you want to be able to manage stress better, you have to learn to solve problems.

I understand that this may not seem like actionable advice. You can't just go out into the world and look for problems to solve (well, you can if you are Spiderman). And you shouldn't go out looking for trouble and bears to cross paths with. Stress management is all about reducing the problems in our life, so how can we practice problem-solving without adding to our stress? Easy, we need to find problems that are not life-threatening or do not have any negative repercussions should we fail. Because, let's face it, we are talking about a need to develop our nonexistent or underdeveloped skills. We are going to fail a few times.

There are problems all around us, every day we are faced with a multitude of opportunities for our brain to strategize, we just have to be able to recognize them for what they are. Household chores, for example. How do I solve the problem of my living room being a complete mess? I can problem solve where to put things so that they aren't scattered about, alleviating the problem of clutter. I can organize drawers, fold clothing, run the vacuum, load the dishwasher, and even make the bed. All of these represent simple problems I can solve to give my brain some practice. These are pretty easy problems to solve too, and will likely end up in a victory, giving you a sense of accomplishment (unless you are trying to fold that fitted bottom sheet, that seems to be an infinite source of stress—I'd rather burn the damn thing). These activities also reduce my stress by making my space seem more comfortable, and some people find that the act of cleaning or organizing helps them relieve stress from other areas of life. Sarah is one of these people, so I always make sure I leave her a little extra to take care of, you know . . . for her mental health. And to Alyssa, if you are reading this when you are older, the reason your mother and I ask you to clean your room is for your brain development. Now pick up them damn toys!

Puzzles are great mental exercise: mazes, crossword puzzles,

Sudoku, brainteasers, trivia, whatever your preference. They provide simple, safe, repercussion-free ways to develop the part of your brain that figures stuff out. Nobody is going to maul you to pieces if you get a word search wrong. Plus, they are problems you can practice solving that don't require having access to other people. Anyway, if you do have people in your life, strategy games like checkers, chess, cards, and Scrabble are also helpful. Some smartphone apps can be great sources of mental exercise and I always have at least one strategy game on my phone. Then again, I could just be rationalizing my phone addiction.

The point is to challenge our brain, repeatedly, until we develop mastery over that level of challenge. Then to step it up a bit. It's like going to the gym to work out your biceps—maybe you start by doing reps with a ten-pound weight, but after a few workouts that weight no longer provides the same quality workout and you increase to fifteen or twenty pounds. Alyssa enacts this process with her toys, moving from one to another.

The same concept applies to your brain. For example, once you have mastered Tetris, maybe you can find a new challenge. I grew up playing Tetris in the arcade, where eventually I got so good that one quarter could last me ten minutes. I've played it on almost every platform since, including every generation of my phone. When I get to a point where I no longer find it challenging, I move on to another game. If you haven't looked, you might be surprised at how many puzzle games are available for mobile use. At this stage in my life, I mainly use them to keep my mind busy when I'm bored, but for people who are actively trying to develop their cognitive skills there are a ton of similar apps and gadgets available.

Speaking of Tetris, one of the things that Sarah does to cope with stress is clean and organize. Over the years, she has become a master organizer, and every time we pack for the road (which is extremely frequent for us) she demonstrates her prowess with a game of "Car Tetris" in which she knows no peer. Man, what I have seen her manage to fit into our hatchback would astonish Robert Ripley.

On another note, pun definitely intended, a few months ago, Sarah noticed that nobody was playing the piano in our home. That may not have been an obvious problem, but it was one that she set out to solve anyway. And in doing so, she helped keep that prefrontal cortex of hers that I love so much all nice and strong. The lesson? If you don't see any problems that need to be addressed and your prefrontal cortex could use a boost, create problems to solve.

One thing that you should understand from this advice is that I am not saying that if you solve a bunch of puzzles you will suddenly be able to face down a bear or remain calm in traffic. There is a *huge* difference in the skill set needed to solve those problems. However, I am saying that stressful events are problems that need to be solved, and the better your brain is at solving problems, the more likely it is react to the next one as if it is something that can be solved. In other words, the more confidence you have in your abilities, the less your reactions will be influenced by feeling stressed.

AND NOW, GILLIGAN, BEFORE WE GET OFF THIS ISLAND, HOW ABOUT SOMETHING FOR OL' SKIMMER?

- If we wish to improve our stress management, we should also develop our problem-solving skills.

- Problem-solving skills can be improved by mastering any challenge that requires strategizing.

Finally, let me add that problem-solving skills, like most acquired functions of the brain, have to be maintained. Again think about the muscle analogy and what happens to them when you stop working out. You don't want to put all that effort into developing your cortex just to have it go the way of your high school Spanish. The phrase "use it or lose it" refers to this phenomenon. As a college student in Texas, I was quick to pick up Spanish and even toured across Mexico during my time off, all the while speaking what I am sure was Spanish. Now, after having moved a few times and not having many opportunities to practice, I sometimes mess up my order at Taco Bell. I'm kidding, of course I order in English, but this is another reason it is important to challenge ourselves and learn new things throughout our lifespan.

You may get to a point where life is pretty comfortable and fewer problems naturally present themselves. For example, other than being fabulously wealthy, I can't think of a lifestyle more comfortable than retirement: the benefits kick in and you get to draw a paycheck just for continuing to breathe. That sounds like living the dream for me, but a lot of retirees develop depression and experience cognitive decline. Almost all of their mental activity was focused on whatever they did for a living, and now their responsibilities include watching *Matlock* reruns and making sure their recliner doesn't float away. My parents retired not too long ago and are always doing what they can to stay busy. My mother has learned new crafts, like basket weaving, and my father has taken on new projects or found things to tinker with in the garage, like his motorcycle. Having an abundance of free time, they also like to travel to exotic, unusual places in the world. Places like Denver, which is super exotic, to visit their granddaughter while her dad writes a book.[53]

Fostering Resilience in Children

When I was growing up, both my parents displayed high levels of resilience. My father was in the military long enough to serve in and survive two wars and my mother, well, she had to deal with him. Resilience may be partially hereditary, but only about half can be attributed to genetic factors. That is the so-called "nature" side of the nature vs. nurture distinction. The other half comes from a combination of nurture and circumstance.

One of the most common questions people have for me when I speak about stress management is "How do we raise resilient children?" I always tell them the same thing: Modeling. How do you teach a child how to walk? How do you teach them how to hold a fork? How do you teach them how to strike a pose and hold it long enough to have their photo taken a few hundred times? Yup, modeling. Now work it!

---

53 By the way, I recently took my daughter into the lab for analysis. As it turns out, she is:

80 percent breast milk

10 percent macaroni and cheese

10 percent candy from Grandma and Grandpa

The best, and most important, way to raise resilient children is to be resilient in their presence. Period. When you blow up and overreact to traffic, think of that person sitting in the car seat behind you and the lessons they are learning. Any behavior that we display in front of our children gets absorbed by the little sponge inside their heads, and all of it has the potential to become part of the way they interact with the world. To our amusement, for months Alyssa has been holding anything cell phone-sized up to her head as if she is having a conversation. Sarah and I find this particularly interesting because we hardly ever use our phones to talk on them. Who does that anymore? Even crazier is when she picks up a rotary phone and pretends to dial. If a child can pick up such an obscure behavior, just imagine what else is sinking into that brain.

Children look to us, not just for guidance, but for examples on how to live and how to handle the different situations they might encounter. If we want our children to grow up to be able to handle whatever life throws at them, then we need to be able to handle whatever life throws at us. I am not saying that we can't let our children see us stress or lose our temper, but they need to see when it is appropriate. They need to learn the difference between bears and unicorns. If they see us freak out, get angry, get upset, fight, yell, or socially withdraw every time something doesn't go our way, then we shouldn't be surprised when they struggle with life as adults.

If we want our children to grow up ready and equipped with the tools for life (and what parent wouldn't), we have to model good problem-solving, as well as healthy coping techniques, like taking time out for ourselves, participating in hobbies, exercise, and socializing. It is important for them to observe us setting boundaries, being flexible, managing expectations of others, and challenging ourselves. You know, all of the things that make us healthy.

Obviously if we want to instill a sense of resilience in our children, we should learn to manage stress ourselves. However, if we don't handle stress well and want a better life for our kids, we need to fake it. Yes, fake it like your ex used to. Fake it for your children. If you are unable to suppress your reactions, at least try to hold them in. Keep your expressions of anger or worrisome thoughts to yourself as much as you can in the presence of your little sponge-brain offspring. Fake it until *they* make it.

Both of my parents were very resilient but my mother was, and still can be, a bit of a worrier. Somehow not only did I grow up without developing this habit, but I really had no idea she worried so much until I was well into adulthood. Early in my career as a public speaker I started discussing worry as a behavior that contributes to anxiety and stress, and the first time my mom saw me speak, she told me that when my brother and I were younger, she used to worry about us all the time. She must have realized the need to keep it to herself because I never knew. She told me about when we lived in upstate New York, in the town of Plattsburgh, and how I would ride my bike into the undeveloped woods near our house. Every time I would head off, she would give me a time to return home and the entire time I was out she would worry about me. I vaguely remember the woods; there were some really cool trails back there, but they must have been near a busy highway. She would imagine all the terrible things that could happen to me. If I was late, she would worry that I got hit by a car and that I was lying dead in a ditch somewhere. What a terrible thing to imagine, but she kept it from me and I would ride home blissfully and completely unaware of her turmoil, ultimately growing up without developing the habit of worrying.

To be fair, now that I am also a parent thoughts of worry do cross my mind occasionally, but they are never something that I hold in my head very long. Check back with me once Alyssa starts riding a bike.

My brother, Jon, and I developed our stress-management skills partly thanks to the environment our parents created for us. Perhaps it was intentional or maybe it was just because they were already resilient and happy themselves, but they raised us in a manner that allowed for our respective personalities to flourish. They never imposed a strict dogma on us or insisted that we follow a particular direction in life. I know so many people who were pushed into activities they did not want or careers they did not choose, but not my brother and me. We were allowed, and encouraged, to pursue multiple interests throughout our lives. The one thing they would always say was that we could do whatever we wanted as long as we were happy; that was pretty much their motto. And trust me, my brother and I put that motto to the test. We were really a couple of underachieving goofballs and yet they were always proud of us. I think they did okay too, raising us. Today, my brother and I aren't Nobel Prize winners or captains of industry, but we aren't total embarrassments either.

I hope that Sarah and I can raise our daughter to be as resilient as my parents raised me to be.

Among the many gifts my parents gave my brother and me was the ability to solve problems. When I was still in college, I was exposed to the Baumrind theory of parenting styles.[54] According to the theory, parents can be categorized based on how much they require their child to adhere to rules and structure, and how responsive they are to their child's needs. A child can develop problems if they are raised without structure or neglected. With regard to resilience, I like to think of successful parenting in terms of problem-solving.

Imagine what would happen to an individual's ability to solve problems if every time they encountered some difficulty, somebody else swooped in and solved their problem for them. Without opportunities to practice problem-solving, they would likely grow up deficient in that regard. Or imagine what would happen if they were consistently shielded from adverse situations and never encountered any problems to solve. Although fortunate, I suppose, they too would likely grow up with a deficiency in problem-solving skills. Nobody wants their kids to suffer or experience pain, but there is value in working through difficulties. There is value in having to deal with adversity. Stepping in or shielding our children may help keep them out of harm's way, but it could have long-term consequences.

I will never forget the day my daughter first walked up stairs without any assistance. We were in New York City at a Central Park playground. There was a really cool structure with a slide and she set her sights on it immediately. She had been practicing

---

54 Diana Baumrind, "Child Care Practices Anteceding Three Patterns of Preschool Behavior," *Genetic Psychology Monographs* 75, no. 1 (1967): 43–88.

Fostering Resilience in Children

stairs for a bit before then, but always needed help or resorted to crawling. On this day, we watched as she got up and kept going all the way to the top of the slide. It was such a cool thing to watch. Having that memory to hold onto means that I will probably never forget this other family that was at the playground at the same time. There were two parents and a toddler, just like the three of us. We find that parents almost always ask each other the age of their offspring, as if making mental comparisons on their own child's progress, and their son was a little more than two years old, about eight months older than Alyssa.

What made this encounter memorable, other than Alyssa's accomplishment, was the overprotective nature of the kid's mother. From the ground level of the park, she loudly barked orders up to her son's father at the top of the slide. (Side note, there are many things I miss from living in New York, but stereotypically loud, nasal people are not one of them.) She shouted that their son was not allowed to go down the slide by himself, an opinion that the father apparently did not share. They shouted back and forth, from the ground to the top of the slide; meanwhile, Alyssa had managed to climb the stairs completely unaccompanied, make it to the top of the slide, and move past the father and son to go down on her own, proudly smiling the entire time. Once she got to the bottom, she happily ran back to the stairs to start all over again. The father even used Alyssa as an example, pleading his case to let their two-year-old son go down the slide on his own. She acquiesced, and their son appeared frightened as he sat down on the slide to head down by himself. The mother in turn ran over to the base of the slide to catch him as soon as he made it down and the three of them moved on to another part of the playground. The slide wasn't even that fast.

I have heard some educational professionals refer to people like that kid's mother as a "helicopter mom," implying that they are always hovering over the child, ready to assist.[55] I love that term, it really resonates with me and fits perfectly into my discussion on problem-solving. As I see it, helicopter parents are stepping in to solve their children's problems, and there is some research that suggests this parenting style can have long-term negative effects with regard to preparing the child for adulthood. For example, college-aged children of helicopter parents have been shown to have a greater tendency toward depression.[56] Successfully going up stairs and down a slide at a playground is not a significant problem, although it comes with a potential for injury, but solving it does help a growing mind develop. I don't know anything about that family from the park other than what I observed in that encounter, but I think about the look of pride on my daughter's face that day and the look of fear on that poor kid. Those could be the foundations of later personality characteristics.

We try to give our daughter enough freedom to explore and make mistakes, but she knows we are never far away when she needs us. As a result (we like to think we've had some influence),

---

55 A term attributed to Foster Cline and Jim Fay. For more, check out their book: Foster Cline and Jim Fay, *Parenting with Love and Logic: Teaching Children Responsibility* (Illinois: Tyndale House, 2006).

56 Holly H. Schiffrin et al., "Helping or Hovering? The Effects of Helicopter Parenting on College Students' Well-Being," *Journal of Child and Family Studies* 23, No. 3 (April 2014): 548–557.

at barely a year and a half, she never backs down from a challenge. Later that evening in New York, Sarah and I took Alyssa to Times Square because that's what you do with a baby in Manhattan. On our way, we encountered a large subway grate. If you've never been to New York City, first of all, go! Second, you may not know that there are ventilation ducts from the subway system that open at the pavement. They allow air to escape the subway system below, relieving pressure and sometimes kicking up Marilyn Monroe's skirt. From an average person's perspective, it is just a grate in the sidewalk where the worst thing you can imagine happening is dropping your keys, but to a baby new to the city, it could look like a free-fall drop into what is surely a pit full of alligators. The three of us approached the grate holding hands, and two of us thought nothing of it. As soon as we got to the edge, Alyssa refused to take another step. The depth below frightened her, so we altered our course around it. The next one we encountered was in Times Square itself, and this time Alyssa led us to the edge. As if she was testing the waters, she stuck one foot out onto the grate and then withdrew. She did it again. Having established that she was not likely going to plummet to her death, she walked out a few steps and came back. She then walked out a few more steps and came back. Finally, she took both Sarah and me by the hand and dragged us out on the grate and danced around triumphantly. After a while, we had to drag her off of it. This is a girl who knows how to face her fears, and *that* behavior is something to foster.

AND TO REALLY HELP DRIVE THE POINT HOME:

- The best way to teach a child how to handle stress is to model resilient behaviors in their presence and try to keep our worry or anger to ourselves.

- Allow children an opportunity to solve their own problems. Provide assistance and support, but give them a chance to attempt things on their own, and the opportunity to fail.

As a parent, I find that it is really hard to let kids just be kids. Sarah and I have to pick our battles; we want to keep our child safe but we also want her to have the freedom to get hurt (just not too badly). It is a tough line to balance.

One of the things that I suspect contributed to my brother's and my resilience was more circumstantial than a function of child-rearing, but it most likely helped us develop our problem-solving skills. As I've mentioned, we grew up in a military home. Our father spent his career in the United States Air Force and it afforded us a great deal of benefits; however, his livelihood also meant that we moved more frequently than most people. About every four years we found ourselves in a different city. In fact, before I turned eighteen, our family lived in three different countries: the United States of America, Germany, and Florida.

Moving around so much has its disadvantages. Especially in those days before the internet, it was hard to establish long-term friendships, the kind you make in childhood that allow you to have a full set of groomsmen at your wedding. It was impossible to grow any roots or feel connected to the larger community. However, the life experiences alone more than made up for any shortcomings of the lifestyle. By the time I entered high school, I had already been all over Europe and exposed to so many more things than most kids my age.

Probably the most significant advantages to moving around frequently as a child were related to our problem-solving skills. Every new environment brings new challenges that must be overcome, and as a child I had to learn how to solve a lot of problems with each duty assignment. Every four years, I had to learn the layout of a new home, a new neighborhood, and a new community. I had to make a new set of friends and get to know a new school with all new teachers and very different cultures. Moving to Alabama, I remember learning about a thing called "po'boys," which suspiciously looked a lot like something we called "sandwiches" in upstate New York. Moving back to New York, I learned that people from Alabama were thought to have banjos on their knees for some reason. And at least one time, I had to learn what it meant to get by in a foreign country and learn to speak an entirely new language. Each time we were relocated, my young world was shaken up and I was given a whole bunch of brand-new problems to solve. Sometimes I was successful, and other times it didn't work out so well, but over my lifetime I became damn good at solving problems.

I should point out that this is probably not a source of practical advice for most people. You want to raise resilient children? Move every four years! Yeah, right.

But what we can do is recognize the potential advantages of shaking things up a bit. We don't have to change cities or countries all the time, but we do need to change our experiences. The more we experience, the more our brain learns to overcome and cope with the problems it encounters. Encourage your child to try out a sport for a while, then maybe learn a musical instrument, then learn to paint or research a subject of interest. By the way, that's good advice at any age. I moved around a lot as a child and I feel that lifestyle helped contribute to my resilience. Let me give you an example of how that helped me.

I wrote the following story about fifteen years ago, about an experience I had at least fifteen years before that. Aside from appearing in a tiny zine back in 2004, this is the first time it is being published.[57] Thinking back on my life, I have always felt it was a good example of how I overcame the challenges, both literally and metaphorically, of a frequently changing environment.

> I was just barely settling into my sophomore year of high school when my life was moved from the New York City area to a rural community outside Austin, Texas. Raised with a city sensibility and a love of all things urban (I actually took a class called "Big Apple Studies"), suffice it to say I didn't quite fit in. The culture shock could have registered on the Richter scale.
>
> I was a punk city kid in a school of painted-on Wranglers, shit-kicking boots, wide-brimmed hats, and long, flowing dusters. In a word: Texans.
>
> Sometime during my second week there, my homeroom teacher read a list of names, all meaningless to me, of the students who were going to represent the sophomore class in the upcoming spirit week competitions for homecoming. After listening to a boring read-through and watching my

---

57 The story was originally written for an underground zine that had an extremely limited circulation in Pittsburgh, Pennsylvania. The version presented here has been edited slightly.

classmates high-five one another after every name, she ended the list with a suggestive "and we *still* don't have a sophomore signed up for the jalapeño-eating contest."

Well, how about that? Eating was something I was pretty good at. I'd never had a *hallo-peen-o* before, but, seriously, how bad could it be? I raised my hand and had the homeroom teacher sign me up to eat jalapeños for the sophomore class. As soon as my name was committed to paper, I suddenly found myself in a press conference fielding questions from all the cowboys and Mexicans in my class. "Dude, you sure you can handle it?" "Ain't they got peppers in New York?" "You know they're hot right?" "*Son muy calientes!*"

That homeroom discussion was the last I heard of the contest for the rest of the week. I went back to living an outsider's life of relative anonymity. I went to my classes, navigating the now-familiar halls and unpaved roads that led to the "temporary" buildings out back that housed the art rooms where I spent a lot of my free time. Nearby, students were grooming livestock for competition and most others were getting excited about homecoming, sporting the school colors and practicing whatever they had to contribute. I noticed the girls started walking around with ridiculously Texas-sized mums pinned to their shirts, dragging trails of ribbons and charms behind them. I didn't feel any school spirit, I didn't care about the sophomore class at all, but damned if I wasn't going to eat me some jalapeños . . . .

As it turned out, Texas homecomings are a big deal. Huge, in fact. Each day was a celebration not only within the school but also in the community. Parents, alums, dropouts, and all sorts of people seemed to show up to the events of spirit week. I was amazed as I looked up at the sea of faces assembled in the gym when I took my position for the contest.

To my left was the freshman: a short, rotund, dark-skinned Mexican kid stuffed into tight western clothes. To my right was the junior: a tall, pale-skinned, red-necked cowboy decked out from hat to heels, including a giant rodeo belt buckle that strained to hold back his massive beer belly. Looking back, it seems odd that a high school student would have a beer gut, but that body type seemed fairly common at my school. The senior was standing to my far right and was less memorable than the others; just a goof-off that didn't seem to be much competition.

The rules were simple: each of us would be given a bowl of peppers and then we would have sixty seconds to eat as many as we could. For each pepper we downed, we would save the stem and the person with the most stems at the end of the minute would win. A cakewalk, I was sure.

The judges then opened up an industrial-sized can of giant ass-kicking jalapeños and proceeded to dump a bowl full of the little bastards in front of each of us. I got my first whiff of the fumes from the can and as I felt the chemical burn in my nose, I realized that I had inadvertently signed up for some serious punishment. Hell, I was someone who considered salt a spice and the most intense flavor I'd ever experienced up until then was probably ketchup. Yet there I was, an out-of-place New Yorker, standing between two intense iron-stomached southwestern eating machines, about to subject myself to gastrological torture for the sake of a sophomore class I didn't care about in a school where I didn't fit in.

"*Go!*"

The start of the contest caught me by surprise, but I quickly grabbed my first jalapeño by the stem and shoved it into my mouth. I bit the end and tried to swallow it whole, thinking that if none of the juice escaped onto my tongue, I'd be okay, but the pepper was too big for that. I bit it into two and swallowed both halves along with the burning juice, trying hard to shuffle my tongue and all of its sensitive taste buds to the side of my mouth and away from the poisonous fluid I had just released. As my right hand lowered the remaining stem into my empty bowl of completes, my left hand quickly stuffed my mouth with another.

My plan seemed to be working. As long as I got them down my throat with minimal contact on my tongue, the peppers weren't that bad. I broke out in a sweat, spilled juice all over my shirt, and felt nauseous as I frantically stuffed pepper after pepper into my face, but at least my mouth wasn't on fire. What's more, I seemed to be keeping pace with my competitors. One after another I swallowed whole jalapeños, sans stems, and did what I could to ignore my increasing level of discomfort.

As the clock ticked, I could feel a burn creeping into my mouth. Starting with a match and a little kindling, it soon progressed to a full three-alarm fire just behind my gums. It took everything I had to keep myself from crying as I continued my regimen of force-feeding.

"... and ... *Stop!*"

I was so relieved to reach the end of one of the longest sixty seconds of my teenage life. After the contest, I was spitting flames, which I tried in vain to douse with water as the judges counted up each contestant's stems. I stood there, sweating in agony as I noticed the others didn't seem to be as affected by the peppers as I was. Figures.

When the final counts were announced, the judges determined that I had eaten twenty-seven full jalapeños in a minute. I won. Hooray for the sophomore class. The Mexican guy came in second, followed by the cowboy, and neither had eaten anywhere near my number.

After the contest, I had to go clean up and arrived late to my homeroom class, where I was greeted with a round of genuine, enthusiastic applause. And it didn't stop there. For the rest of the day I was congratulated, patted on the back, high-fived, and otherwise acknowledged by my new peers. I made new friends and found myself being invited to all sorts of parties and events. Sure, I felt ill, and my mouth was still in pain, but for the first time since leaving New York, I felt accepted.

It wasn't a rodeo, but I had competed with Texans, in one of their games, and won. In just sixty seconds I had made the transition from outsider to cowboy and all it took was a few hot peppers.

Thirty-something years later, looking back, I wouldn't say this single event changed my life or was a precise turning point for me, but perhaps it was a part of something greater. I fell in love with Texas, and stayed in Austin after high school to attend college. I've assimilated some of the cowboy culture into my life. As I'm writing this, I'm wearing cowboy boots and Wrangler jeans, a collection of felt cowboy hats hangs on my coatrack, and I even listen to a little bit of country music.

Moreover, this story shows how a lifetime of changing environments and different experiences helped me adapt to my new surroundings. As a kid faced with the problems of adjusting to a new school, I saw an opportunity and I took it. Ultimately, this event probably helped plant the seed of what would later influence my life a great deal. I developed a taste for public attention (and spicy food), and this contributed to my career as a professor, presenter, and ultimately an entertainer. And, to this day, I still like jalapeños.

AND FOR THOSE OF YOU WHO SKIPPED THE JALAPEÑOS:

- The more we experience, the more our brain also learns to solve problems.

8

Practicing
Positive Thinking

B y now some of you might be thinking, "So stress is all in your head, right?" Now, sure, some stress is a product of our thoughts, but remember, there are real stressors in the world: attacking bears, vans breaking down in Mexico, adjusting to new high schools, or worse. Sometimes life deals us shitty circumstances. Sometimes you can't do anything about those circumstances. But you can change how they affect you.

The only part of your brain that you have voluntary control over is the activity of your prefrontal cortex, your thoughts. Your thoughts influence both your behaviors and your emotions, and it is important to understand this in order to make any changes. If that sounds really simple to you, that is because it is. The key to making some pretty significant changes in our lives is to adjust the way we think. We tend to think that our lives, our problems and issues, are extremely complicated and overcoming them requires a complicated solution. Making changes can be simple, it just isn't easy.

Stating that something is simple is not the same thing as claiming it is easy. And it is important to understand the difference. So many of our problems have simple solutions, but they are difficult to implement. For example, one of the most common questions people have for me, other than those that relate to stress, is if I have any advice on how to lose weight. Which is ironic, if you could see me. I am not exactly the poster child for weight loss, but I have studied it quite a bit and know a lot about it. Sure, there are tons of special diets to follow and a plethora of books to explain them to you—hell, if this gets shelved in the self-help section, they might even be my neighbors. However, whatever those books are selling you, the key to losing weight is simple: eat less and exercise more. But that would make for a really short book. Eating less and exercising more is not complicated, but it is far from easy and maybe that is the true value of those books: each of them offers its own way for you to eat less and exercise more.

Similarly, people ask me how to quit smoking, and the answer is simple: stop putting cigarettes in your mouth. Yeah, but how do I do that? I don't know, maybe stop buying them? This isn't a book on smoking cessation. The point being that 100 percent of all smokers know exactly how to quit smoking, it is just implementing that knowledge that is really, really hard. People also ask me how to stop drinking or doing drugs . . . do we really need more examples here? The answers are simple, carrying out the answer is what's difficult. Which explains why, as someone who not only knows the key to how to lose weight, but has also studied the brain mechanisms behind appetite quite extensively, I still carry extra body weight.[58] A seminar attendee once asked me for advice on how to lose weight, and I told her what I always say, "Eat less and exercise more," to which she replied, "Is there anything else? I really like eating and I hate exercise!"

People ask me how to live happier lives, and I tell them to manage their stress. Managing stress and becoming more resilient is a simple answer, but it definitely ain't easy. Among the things that I have discussed so far, we need to learn to tell the difference between an actually threatening situation and one that is just annoying or inconvenient, feel as if we are in control, and develop our problem-solving skills. Those are all relatively simple lessons to learn and yet, they all take work and a lot of practice over time. There is no quick fix that will magically bestow upon us overnight the ability to remain calm, no matter how badly we want it. But wouldn't it be nice? It would be wonderful if there was some magical secret, but for weight loss, stress resilience, and most forms of change, the answer is staring us in the face, it just isn't pretty. Unfortunately, it's the only one that swiped right.

Although it takes time and effort to become resilient, the good news is that there are some relatively easy practices we can incorporate into our lives to help us get there. I refer to this as the act of practicing positive thinking. In this section, I will discuss techniques that can help minimize stressful thinking and at the same time increase resilient thoughts. These are some mental

---

58 Although at the time of writing this, I am happy to say that, even after Thanksgiving and helping the baby finish off her Halloween candy, I am carrying thirty-seven pounds less than I was last year.

exercises we can engage to give that left side of our prefrontal cortex a little extra activity.

THREE WAYS POSITIVE THINKING CAN HELP YOU BECOME MORE STRESS RESILIENT ARE:

1. Teaching you to become more optimistic.

2. Teaching you to be more appreciative of what you have.

3. Increasing your appreciation of humor.

See? Simple and easy! Okay, let me explain these in more detail.

First, do something with me and quickly imagine what life might be like in the future. Do you imagine a utopian world that has solved all of the pressing issues such as overpopulation, resource distribution, waste management, pollution, and transportation? Or do you imagine a dystopian future where these have become so problematic as to make the world practically unlivable? In other words, is the future you imagine more like *Star Trek* or *Wall-E*? If you imagine a bright future, you probably tend to be optimistic, and if your image of the future seems bleak, well then, you probably don't. Personally, I think the future is bright. I recognize that there are some serious issues facing us, such as climate change and economic inequality, but I also know that as a species we are extremely resilient. We have survived plagues, world wars (two of them, I hear!), global economic depressions, the release of *The Emoji Movie*, and all sorts of natural disasters, and each time we come out swinging like a collective Captain America saying, "I can do this all day!" I don't know how we will solve our problems, but I am confident that somehow some of us will solve some of them. This point of view would put me in the optimist category. I know plenty of people who have less faith, believing that some of the damage we have done is irreversible or that human nature is self-destructive and we are doomed to experience another *Emoji Movie*.

I have shared with you that I am a happy person. I have also shared that I am a resilient person, and you know that these two things are highly related. Guess where optimism fits in? Well to start, optimistic thinking is positively correlated with happiness. Optimistic people are happier and happy people are more optimistic. Optimistic people are also more resilient, are less affected by stress, and worry less often. All of this should make sense to you in the context of everything I have discussed. Resilience and happiness are a function of the types of thoughts we have and optimism is a way of thinking. So yeah, optimistic thinking contributes to both resilience and happiness. Although I am not the most optimistic person I know, I would definitely label myself an optimist.

Optimism is also a reaction. The brain has a wide range of potential reactions. When we encounter a stimulus, for example a piece of information, we can react to it by putting a positive spin on it, or we can worry about it. Worrying is a form of pessimistic thinking. Depending on which is more frequent, and therefore more likely to be our reaction, we may identify as either an optimist or a pessimist. However, most of us fall somewhere in the middle of that dichotomy, even if we lean to one side more than the other. I should also let you in on a little secret: optimistic people have pessimistic thoughts all the time. The most optimistic people among us are still plagued by negative thoughts, the difference is that they don't dwell on them or ruminate.

I find that people who are prone to worry have a hard time imagining how optimistic thinking can be an alternative, but it is. They often say to me that they feel they have to worry. I always tell them they probably do not, as there are few stimuli that necessitate worry. There are always alternative reactions. For example, a couple of chapters ago I shared how my mother worried about me when I was riding my bike. If I was late, she would worry that I got hit by a car and that I was lying dead in a ditch somewhere. The stimulus in this situation was the realization that it was after my expected return time and I had not yet come home; obviously the reaction was to worry. It might make sense for a parent to worry about their kids, but that isn't the only possible response to that stimulus. An optimistic person might respond to that same stimulus with an entirely different response: "Oh, look at that, my kid is late coming home. You know what, I bet he's out there having a lot of fun. He probably just lost track of time and cell phones haven't been invented yet. He will probably be home soon or when he gets hungry." Same exact stimulus, with two very different responses. You don't have to worry.

Unless the kid is *really* late. Then worry. Or worry whenever, you know your kid better than I do. Sometimes worry is an appropriate response.

If you are prone to worry you probably aren't very optimistic (or happy or resilient), but don't fret (any more than you usually do)—you can become optimistic through practice. And, as I mentioned, it is not that difficult. I want you to imagine the future, only this time imagine that everything has worked out for you exactly as you want it. What does that look like? Be as descriptive as possible. Now write that down in a journal and repeat this exercise again next week, focusing on a different aspect of your life (such as career or relationship). If you did what I asked, and I know that you probably did not (but you should!), what you just did was a version of a task called "the best possible selves activity" originally presented by Dr. Laura King (no relation).[59] This activity, which involves nothing more than writing in a journal once a week, has been shown to increase optimistic thinking.[60]

The best possible selves activity is a simple journaling exercise. You don't have to be a good writer, you don't have to write a lot, and obviously you don't have to accurately predict the future (although that would be super cool if you could). All you have to do is set aside some time on a regular basis to force your brain to think positively about the future. Which, if you are not very optimistic, you may recognize as precisely what your brain is not doing enough of. Actually, you probably don't even need to write, but having the journaling exercise helps focus your thoughts.

- Structured journaling exercises can help us learn to be more optimistic, which in turn can help us manage stress.

Keep in mind that this is not the sort of cure-all that is going to radically turn your life around overnight. If you go into the gym

---

59 Laura A. King, "The Health Benefits of Writing about Life Goals," *Personality and Social Psychology Bulletin* 27, no. 7 (July 2001): 798–807.

60 For a good review, see Paula M. Loveday, Geoff P. Lowell, and Christian M. Jones, "The best possible selves intervention: A review of the literature to evaluate efficacy and guide future research," *Journal of Happiness Studies* 19, no. 2 (February 2018): 607–628.

and you do a single curl, you won't walk out with a giant bicep. You have to do thousands of curls over a long period of time to get that desired outcome, which will look strange because you forgot to work out your other arm. Writing in a journal is not going to make you immediately optimistic, but practicing positive thinking on a regular basis will have an impact on your thinking.

Okay, now let's discuss how we can become more appreciative of what we have. In the past few decades there has been a significant increase in the amount of academic research on happiness. As a result, we now know a lot about what makes some people happier than others and how we can become happier. One behavior that happier people engage in more often than less happy people is expressing positive emotions. Love, for example, is a very positive emotion and most of us feel it for people in our lives. However, not all of us are equally expressive of that emotion. Some rarely tell others how they feel, whereas there are some people who are extremely expressive of positive emotions. We have a word for people like that, we call them "happy."

Remember that our thoughts influence our emotions. To verbally express our love or appreciation for someone else requires that we also put that thought into our head, which in turn makes us happy. In other words, the act of telling someone you love that you love them makes you happier. Now, don't worry if you are unable to commit to something as strong as love. Whether it's love, like, admiration, or appreciation, pretty much any sincere positive emotion expressed to another person can have an impact. We can increase the positive thoughts in our head by being more expressive of our feelings for other people. Of all the advice I give people on a regular basis, this is my favorite. Tell the people you love that you love them more often. Plus, as a bonus, it usually has this really cool side effect of making the other person happier too.

I should emphasize the word "sincere" in the above paragraph. You have to actually mean it. Please don't go out into the world telling a bunch of random strangers that you love them. I am pretty sure that would not provide the desired effect. It is not my intent to inspire a bunch of players.

As much as I advocate expressing our love and gratitude to the people in our lives, there are limits to how often we can express such things before we become annoying. There is such a thing as too much, even when it comes to expressions of positive emotions. Plus, not everyone has people in their lives that they love or appreciate. Maybe you just aren't there yet. Some people are uncomfortable expressing themselves this way, and a recommendation to do so is probably a frightening (and stressful) prospect. Remember, if you are stressing out about being happy, you are doing it wrong. If the very thought of engaging a behavior intended to increase your happiness causes you stress, then you might want to find another activity that promotes positive thinking.

Thankfully, positive psychologists have come up with a few really good alternative activities we can practice. My favorite of these, and the one that I most often recommend to people in my seminars, in consultation, or even in my personal life, is the practice of gratitude journaling. There are different formats, but I prefer the simple act of ending each day by listing three or more things that I am grateful for about that day. Often this is referred to as the "three good things exercise," because what else would you call it?[61] Some people write three things they are thankful for, others prefer to count their blessings each day, but these are just variations of the same theme. Chances are you have already heard of this as it has become super popular. It is commonly recommended by therapists, and openly discussed by celebrities. For example, *Frasier* actor Kelsey Grammer and *Guardians of the Galaxy* actor Chris Pratt engage in gratitude practices.[62] Proud Texan, and Austin's favorite citizen, musician Willie Nelson claimed the practice turned his life around.[63] Actress Emma Watson wrote about her journaling practice, "I love the idea of starting my day by listing three things I'm grateful for. And going to bed thinking about the three amazing things that happened in the day. I'm a big believer in the transformative practice of gratitude."[64] And if Hermione Granger's words aren't enough of an endorsement, Oprah Winfrey herself has been practicing gratitude for over a decade, and, despite her incredibly busy schedule, finds time to write five things a day![65]

Personally, I can't think of an easier way to increase happiness than listing three good things at the end of the day. It barely takes five minutes to do, and the potential return on that time and

---

61 M. E. Seligman et al., "Positive Psychology Progress: Empirical Validation of Interventions," *American Psychologist* 60, no. 5 (2005): 410–421.

62 Janice Kaplan, "What Really Makes Celebrities Grateful?" *Time*, August 18, 2015, https://time.com/4002315/jake-gyllenhaal-gratitude-celebrity/.

63 Willie Nelson and Turk Pipkin, *The Tao of Willie: A Guide to the Happiness in Your Heart* (New York, NY: Penguin, 2007).

64 "Book Club with Emma Watson: The Actor Shares her Ultimate Reading List," *Vogue Australia*, March 8, 2018, http://vst.to/wih77BH.

65 Oprah Winfrey, "What Oprah Knows for Sure about Gratitude," *O: The Oprah Magazine*, November 2012, http://www.oprah.com/spirit/oprahs-gratitude-journal-oprah-on-gratitude.

minimal effort is incredible. All of us, regardless of our circumstances, can find three things to be grateful for each day. Even on the absolute worse days, there are things to appreciate. In fact, it is on those days that this exercise might help us the most, reminding us that despite all the crap we dealt with, there is still good in our lives.

Touring the country as long as I have, I had been recommending this practice to my seminar attendees for years. Then, "gratitude challenges" of some form or another started popping up a lot in my Facebook feed. Usually I would see seven-day challenges, but occasionally the challenge would be for twenty-one or thirty-day periods. When I started seeing this, I immediately recognized its source, and could not help feeling a bit jealous that I didn't come up with the idea myself. What an absolutely brilliant idea! As long as you are going to waste time scrolling through Facebook anyway, you might as well use it to make you happy. You know, in between posting pictures of your food. Or combine it. For some people, Facebook is like: "This is what I had for breakfast . . . This is what I had for lunch . . . This is what I had for dinner . . . Here are three things about today that I am grateful for: breakfast, lunch, and dinner."

It makes sense, really; Facebook is already designed to be used for short journal entries. They may call them "updates" but it is a form of journaling. However, in my opinion, the real advantage of practicing gratitude on Facebook is that it is shared with our family and friends (and that guy you hardly remember from high school but whose friend request you accepted anyway). When you keep a gratitude journal it contributes to your happiness, but when you share that journal publicly you invite a whole additional element.

People provide you feedback, they validate your experiences, and they are inspired to do it on their own.

In my seminars, I started challenging my audience to do this on Facebook, and because I try to practice what I preach, I moved my gratitude posts to my Facebook page. Originally, I intended to simply provide a model of the exercise for people to view, but I found the activity so rewarding I kept it going every day (with very few exceptions) for over three years. In fact, I only stopped the practice when I began writing this book and have every intention of returning to it once I complete the book. Don't get me wrong; I still keep a gratitude journal, I just cut back on social media time to get some work done. In fact, here is my entry for today so you can see how I do it.

THREE THINGS I AM GRATEFUL FOR ABOUT TODAY, DECEMBER 4:

1. The apartment we are renting is in close proximity to several nice parks and playgrounds. I have noticed that winter weather in Denver comes and goes, and today was relatively warm so Alyssa and I spent some time at one of the parks and enjoyed the playground.

2. Sarah found us a great place to stay for our upcoming month in Florida. It is in a rural part of northern Florida and on a working farm complete with all sorts of animals. We are excited because neither of us has lived on a farm before, and it might be a lot of fun for Alyssa.

3. Although he just recently visited Denver with my parents, my brother, Jon, is planning on coming back to Colorado to spend Christmas with us. It will be great to see him and have more family to share the holiday with.

And that's it. I always find it helpful to add a little explanation of why I am grateful for each item on my list. One thing that is important about the exercise is that it is focused on the current day. If you just list three things you are grateful for in general, then every day you will have the same list. For example, one person who took me up on the challenge posted "My health, my husband, my kids" every day. By making it specific to today, you force your brain to reflect on all the positives that you have recently experienced, putting activity into the left side of your prefrontal cortex. And this is the whole point.

By the way, if you haven't guessed it yet I am officially challenging you to do the gratitude challenge on Facebook. For a period of at least seven days, at the end of the day post the three things you are grateful for and then challenge others to do it as well. At the end of that week you may notice that you feel happier. In fact, you may decide to keep doing it beyond the challenge. One of my friends did this for a year, and I still see past attendees post their lists. If it seems like a strange thing to start doing, you can even blame it on me. Do this *only* if you are already on Facebook, please don't sign up for an account because of me. If you have somehow avoided it so far, please continue enjoying what must be a very fulfilling life.

If you are not into social media, please consider this a challenge to start gratitude journaling the old-fashioned way. It is easy to do, does not take a lot of time, and can have a positive impact on your life.

TO SUMMARIZE THIS SECTION FOR THE YOU-KNOW-WHOS:

- Verbally expressing positive emotions, such as love or gratitude, to others can make us happier and in turn help us manage stress.

- Keeping a gratitude journal, specifically listing three things we appreciate about each day, can also make us happier.

Okay, so that covers learning to become more optimistic, and learning to be more appreciative of what you have. The third simple and easy activity I mentioned was to increase your appreciation of humor. I am sure that you know what humor is, but to relate it to the context of what I have discussed here, humor is our brain's ability to recognize a potentially threatening stimulus as amusing or nonthreatening. It involves initially perceiving the stimulus one way, and then immediately reinterpreting it as something else. The brain recognizes this process as humorous.[66] I know that may sound confusing, so let me give you an example.

My favorite joke is an old one that I am sure you have heard before. It is the famous one-liner by Henny Youngman, "Take my wife . . . please." It is a simple joke, and will hopefully help you understand what I mean about how the brain processes humor. The first three words set up the joke, or establish the premise. The phrase "take my wife" signals to your brain that he is about to begin talking about his wife. He pauses for a beat and unconsciously we are now expecting him to continue with a joke about his wife. When he continues with the word "please," it completely changes

---

66 Y. C. Chan et al., "Segregating the Comprehension and Elaboration Processing of Verbal Jokes: An fMRI Study," *NeuroImage* 61, no. 4 (July 2012): 899–906.

the meaning of the sentence and our brain has to immediately reinterpret it. The result of this quick shift in our understanding strikes our brain as funny. Since our brain recognizes that it made a mistake in its initial assumption, and because the situation is nonthreatening, we are amused. I did the same thing early in this book when I said that I recently became a father. This was actually a joke I often tell on stage. When I say, "At the age of forty-five, I became a dad. I know what you are thinking," your mind assumes I will go in one direction, and when I end it with "Babies having babies! This man is too young to have a child!" it changes direction completely.

Most jokes are more complicated than simply adding a word or phrase to the end of a sentence to change its meaning, but I hope that these examples help you see that humor is the result of changing our initial perception of something. Suppose I am hiking a trail in the Rocky Mountains and through the woods I think I see a bear in the distance. Instinctively, I may be immediately filled with fright, as I am unsure if I am going to be attacked or if the bear is just going to ignore me, but then I see it move toward me and as it comes closer into my view, suddenly I realize, *Oh man, that's just my cousin Shawn!* I laugh as my brain realizes its error and feel relief that I am no longer going to get mauled by a bear. Shawn might want to kick my ass when he reads this, but I can take him. Also, you are very hairy, Shawn. It's about time someone said something.

Having a sense of humor means being able to understand things in multiple ways, and this is incredibly helpful in overcoming stress. As I have mentioned, inner areas of our brain may misinterpret a stimulus as a potential threat, thereby engaging our stress response, but our prefrontal cortex has the ability to override this system by thinking differently. I know a guy who wrote an entire book on the mental and physical benefits of humor, but from my perspective this is the exact purpose of humor.[67] It helps keep the brain from becoming unnecessarily stressed. Most theories of humor are consistent with this view as well, whether it is believed to reduce tension or to serve as a defense mechanism. Humor is even used by some other species as a means to help reduce aggression in social settings.[68] There are a lot of benefits of humor, but I believe stress management is the most important.

In addition to redirecting potentially negative brain activity, humor also has the nice benefit of inspiring us to laugh. You have probably heard the phrase "Laughter is the best medicine." It gets tossed around a lot, and people don't put too much thought into it. Because I am a comedian with a degree in psychology and have written a book on this very subject, people often ask me if the saying is true. As much as I would like to say it is, of course it's not. Laughter isn't going to help you beat the flu, it isn't going to cure your toe fungus, and it most certainly is not going to fix your broken arm. However, laughter may help you prevent or recover from cancer,[69] it may help you avoid cardiovascular disease by lowering

---

67 Um, duh. Me, I am talking about me.

68 Charles Darwin, *The Expression of the Emotions in Man and Animals* (New York, NY: Oxford University Press, 2009) and Robert R. Provine, *Laughter: A Scientific Investigation* (New York, NY: Penguin, 2001).

69 Mary P. Bennett et al., "The Effect of Mirthful Laughter on Stress and Natural Killer Cell Activity," *Nursing Faculty Publications: Alternative Therapies* 9, no. 2 (March 2003): 38–45.

your blood pressure,[70] it might help you manage your diabetes,[71] and it will certainly help manage your stress.

Stress is our brain's reaction to threat and it gets us ready for some sort of action. When we stress, cortisol flows through our body, resulting in all sorts of physiological changes. Problems arise when our body starts producing all this potential for action, and has no action to take. However, the physical act of laughing involves an enormous amount of activity across a bunch of different areas. From the electrical activity in the brain as you process the humor, to the facial muscles that make you smile and laugh, to the diaphragm that forces the lungs to inhale and exhale, to the arm and leg muscles that are engaged when you clap and stomp your feet, laughter inspires a tremendous chain of bodily activity. Laughter is a profound release of stress, which reduces cortisol and has the added bonus of making us feel good.

Laughter is not only an expression of our happiness, it also contributes to it. Recall that I briefly described the James-Lange Theory of Emotion, where our brain interprets our emotional state from physiological cues. If our body is smiling, laughing, or clapping, what sort of emotion do you think you will start to experience? I'll give you a hint, it starts with an "H." Yes, you guessed it: hysteria. Duh, happiness. Which is why you can probably understand how happy I was when my daughter started displaying

---

70 Herbert M. Lefcourt, "Humor as a Stress Moderator in the Prediction of Blood Pressure Obtained during Five Stressful Tasks," *Journal of Research in Personality* 31, no. 4 (December 1997): 523–542.

71 Richard S. Surwit and Mark S. Schneider, "Role of Stress in the Etiology and Treatment of Diabetes Mellitus," *Psychosomatic Medicine* 55, no. 4 (1993): 380–393.
See also Keiko Hayashi et al., "Laughter Lowered the Increase in Postprandial Blood Glucose," *Diabetes Care* 26, no. 5 (May 2003): 1651–1652.

an appreciation for humor. At eight months she already laughed a lot and had two really distinct laughs, a "ha ha ha" type that almost sounded as if she was forcing it, and a giggle that sounded much more authentic. Almost a year later her sense of humor seems to be developing nicely. She even tells jokes. Obviously, without the language skills, they are slapstick, but they are jokes nonetheless. The first joke I remember was when the three of us were in the car and she tapped on Sarah's shoulder from her car seat. When Sarah turned around, Alyssa crammed one of her toys into Sarah's mouth and started laughing. I nearly busted a gut I laughed so hard. More recently, she led me by the hand over to my shoes as if encouraging me to take her for a walk. When I reached down to put my shoe on, I noticed one of her toys stuffed inside. As soon as I saw it, she started laughing hysterically. People that make you laugh contribute to your health and happiness. I love my daughter.

So what do you do with this information? Well, I think the most obvious answer is to realize the impact that humor has on stress and engage in humorous activity more often. Joking is a great way to cope with a stressor or diminish the effect it has on us. In fact, a lot of humor comes from negative experiences or dark thoughts. Sitcoms and movies frequently make light of difficult situations, and stand-up comedians bring all sorts of pain to the stage. Humor is a great coping mechanism and learning how to laugh it off can be a helpful skill. Not all of us are equally gifted when it comes to generating humor, but thankfully listening to or watching comedy is also extremely helpful.

NOW TO RECAP FOR THE SKIMMERS:

- Humor is a natural stress-management tool.

- Reevaluating a situation to make a joke can help reduce negative thinking.

- The physical act of laughing reduces stress and stress-related physiological conditions.

I began performing stand-up comedy about a year or two before I became a public speaker. For most of my life, I had wanted to be a comedian, but kept putting it off for one reason or another. When I was a college student in Austin, I used to go to a lot of comedy shows. I really appreciated the local Texan scene and saw the legendary Bill Hicks perform during the recording of his last albums.[72] I saw Ron White early in his career, working the clubs in Austin. The Velveeta Room comedy club, now a staple on the comedy circuit, opened up on 6th Street while I was living there and I went to their shows often enough that I got to know several of the local comedians. They would always encourage me to give stand-up a shot, but for some reason I just did not feel ready. I left Austin for graduate school in New Orleans and then Ohio, where my studies consumed most of my time. After that, I am not sure what kept me off the stage but I do know what finally got me on there: stress.

Eventually I moved to San Francisco and found myself working a job I absolutely hated. It wasn't the company's fault; I was

---

72 This is actually a point of pride for me. I was at the taping of Hicks's album *Arizona Bay* at the Laff Stop in Austin (now the Cap City Comedy Club). I was in the front row and he made fun of my shirt. I shook his hand after the show. Later, when the album was posthumously released, I noticed that at least one point my laugh is clearly audible. He was, and still is, a significant inspiration to me.

just in the wrong environment at the wrong time of my life. I never really connected with my coworkers, and I found my work to be very unfulfilling. The stress of that job took its toll on me and I developed a mild case of depression. Adding additional stress to my life was the cost of living in San Francisco, something that I would have had a hard time affording without continuing to work that job that I hated. Like many people in similar situations, I felt trapped. A friend of mine, also trained in psychology, suggested that I try stand-up comedy and reminded me of my lifelong desire. I signed up for my first open mic the following week. Almost immediately I felt relief from my depression and an elevation in my mood, so I kept with it. A month later, I was performing regularly, laid off from that job, and never happier. Now, before you quit your day job and run off to develop a tight five minutes, understand that comedy is a difficult industry and the odds of being successful are stacked against you. I have attained more success as a public speaker than I probably ever will as a comedian. It requires incredible resilience and very likely another means of support; I don't recommend it as a career option. However, it was exactly the thing I needed at one of the most stressful periods of my life, and I have never looked back. Even tomorrow evening, I am taking time out from working on this book to perform at a local Denver comedy show.

Laughing It Off

Before I get into this section, I just have to mention that this morning after she woke up, she picked out her own clothes for the day *and* put on her own jeans halfway up! I know it may be oversharing, but I am so proud of Sarah.

For a comedian, you might think I would have devoted a lot more real estate in this book to discussing humor. I could go on and on about the benefits of humor but for the purposes of this thing we are doing now, it is enough to say that having a sense of humor and laughing helps relieve stress. Different studies have shown that laughter lowers cortisol and blood pressure, leaving me to conclude that laughter is nature's stress-management system.

Stand-up comedy helped me to overcome one of the most stressful periods of my life, and my sense of humor has helped me through everything I have ever encountered. My sense of humor helped me to adjust to the culture of my new high school in Texas, it later helped me manage my response to having my car broken into repeatedly while living in the French Quarter, and recently it helped me to deal with the headaches of managing the repairs to my condo from fifteen hundred miles away.

When people learn that I am a comedian who also holds a doctorate, they often remark how that is a rare combination. It is rare, and yet I personally know many people who have earned the right to include "Dr." in their stage name, even more when you include those with a Juris Doctorate. There are a lot of famous examples; comedian, actor, and medical doctor Ken Jeong is probably the biggest name to come to mind. I have met a lot of other people with advanced degrees who have chosen to pursue comedy at least part-time or have changed careers completely. That said, it is common for me to be the only doctor in a show. When comedian Dave DeLuca and I ran our show together in Los Angeles, he scheduled the performers and I often served as host. I had not previously met Dr. Laura Hayden, but after she played our stage and had us all laughing hysterically, I became a fan. This is her story, and as it turns out, we had more in common than we realized.[73]

Comedy saved my career as a physical therapist.

I was one year into my career as a physical therapist. I had landed a dream job straight out of school in an outstanding orthopedic sports clinic, a position rarely acquired by a newbie. But one year into a profession that took an arduous eight years of college and hundreds of hours of internships my job was killing me.

No medical school or program that I know of teaches you how to properly deal with the emotional, mental, physical, and even spiritual drain treating patients can have on your psyche. I was burnt out one year into my career, not good since it would take a decade to pay off my student loans.

I waited tables forever because I went to school forever. At

73 Shared with me via email in December 2018.

last count I have six college degrees and transcripts from nineteen universities. No one smart should ever follow my example. I am good at *Jeopardy*, however. I began waiting tables early in my college career for two reasons: first, to get over my debilitating shyness, and second, to make more money than working sales in a sad retail store in a very past-its-prime mall. All my regular restaurant costumers would often remark that I was funny. Honestly, I have never thought of myself as funny. I think I have a quick mind and I'm honest, which has led to a few gems on the restaurant floor.

My graduate program for physical therapy required that we give an enormous amount of presentations. They wanted all of us to be effective communicators, or at least that is the BS they sold us. In retrospect, I actually think it was good training. My classmates were always excited when I gave my presentations because they were funny. Once again, I was not trying to be funny while talking about spinal meningitis, or some other equally unfunny subject, but it happened. Anyhow, my amusing presentations led my graduating class to nominate me to give the commencement speech. Again, I was not trying to be funny, just not boring, because it is notoriously a very boring speech. "We would like to thank the faculty . . . blah blah blah." Meanwhile the entire audience just wishes it was over so they could go eat celebration cake. Really, the only reason anyone goes to a graduation is for the cake. I was terrified, but the speech was a hit; I had to pause several times because people were laughing so hard. Afterward, the many accolades signaled to me that I was a natural up there. Little do they know I threw up twice before, the curse of every extreme introvert.

Long story short, every new year instead of giving up something, because I can never manage to stop eating, drinking, or swearing, I try something new. I flipped a coin to decide if I should take a stand-up class or sailing lessons. Heads came up so it was stand-up. I just planned to take the class, do the showcase, and move on with my life, but stand-up fed something in me that I didn't even know was missing. It started as a lark, but every time I did a show, I felt better. After work I was so exhausted, both mentally and physically. On some days I could barely walk to my car, but somehow, I would drag myself to an open mic, watch comedy, and perform. I would leave the comedy venue at midnight feeling better than I had at seven in the evening. This happened over and over again. Comedy literally pulled me out of a severe case of burnout.

Since I'm a big nerd and the effect of laughter was so profound in my life, I started doing research on the healing aspects of laugher. Surprisingly enough, this led me back to college. I went back and got my PhD and my dissertation was on the healing aspects of laughter as it pertains to caretaker stress and burnout.

Comedy has had the most profound positive effect on my life. It has now allowed me to perform in thirty-one countries and I have met amazing people and friends. And it saved my physical therapy career. You don't need to read my 782-page dissertation, I will sum it up for you—comedy is good for you, really good for you. Go out and laugh, your health actually depends on it.[74]

---

74 Laura Hayden is a physical therapist, comedian, speaker, and author, among other things. You can find more about her at www.laurahayden.com.

Obviously, I know from experience that burnout is absolutely terrible, and healthcare professions such as physical therapy, nursing, and medicine have some of the highest rates. Burnout is a form of work-related stress that can take its toll on our mental and physical health just like any other form of stress. What makes burnout a bit more challenging is that most people really need their jobs, so they can't simply remove that source of stress. They feel trapped. They can't run, and they can't fight, so they very often do nothing (freeze), which makes the situation worse and worse. For those of us with an advanced education or specialized skill set, the stress is amplified because we feel that we have invested so much time and energy into our career, we need it to pay off out of a lack of options. Having suffered from burnout at a few points in my life, I often speak out about the harm it causes. Anti-burnout, I know, how edgy! I'm all about pushing the envelope.

Most of us have to work, and as long as we do, hopefully we can enjoy stimulating, rewarding, and maybe personally fulfilling careers. However, not all jobs are great, and sometimes we are going to have to take a position that might fall short of our dream job just to make ends meet. If a job can't be great, at a bare minimum it should not make you sick. I think it is a reasonable expectation, and yet so many of us work jobs that are doing just that. Imagine a situation where a person suffering burnout develops depression. That depression is going to impact that person's productivity, as well as their life outside of work. Thankfully there are potential treatments for depression. Imagine that this person seeks out therapy. Perhaps they are prescribed an antidepressant to help their situation. Now, they are taking medicine to manage their illness brought on by their crappy job so that they can continue working the same crappy job. But now, they really can't quit the job because they need the insurance that pays for the pills that help them do the job that's causing the depression! Obviously life is not this simple, but you see how some people can get trapped in a vicious unhealthy cycle.

Breaking a cycle is not easy, but for Laura and me, our sense of humor helped and even led us into some really interesting careers. Becoming a comedian is not a viable solution for everyone, but even if you just unwind after hours with a little fun, humor can help take the edge off a crappy job.

I first met Conor Kellicutt in San Francisco. He was already a well-established headlining comedian when I hit the scene. Because he was higher than me in the comedy food chain, we did not find ourselves on the same shows very often, but I would see him around. One of the professional comedy clubs in the city, the Punch Line, had a weekly showcase of local comedians. For established acts, it was a great place to get in a fun set and for the newbies, it was a weekly opportunity to network and learn through observation. When I started out, I attended every week I could, just to see the show. Conor was a regular performer and I really enjoyed his style. We eventually connected on social media, and although it has been years since we last saw each other in person, I enjoy keeping up with his posts. Over the years, he has never failed to make me laugh, even when he experienced an unimaginable tragedy. This is his story.[75]

---

75 Shared with me via email in November 2018.

As a comedian I have made humor a huge part of my life and have used it extensively to get through tough times. As the class clown, I used it to deflect the negative attention of bad grades. In a family with alcoholism and divorce I used it to escape horrible moments. I even joked my way out of many fistfights.

At one point in my life, I had two kids and a wife and was losing my house. At that time, doing actual stand-up kept me going; telling jokes to people about how hard life was seemed to be relieving stress for me and them. It kept me from breaking and going insane from the incredible financial stress.

I have often used humor to cut tension and relieve stress. However, there was one time a friend used it to help me when I was in the worst place in my life and I couldn't find the funny myself.

In 2011, Cindy, my love, my wife of fourteen years, the mother of our two children, Shane, eleven, and Hanna, thirteen, died suddenly. I could never have imagined what that would be like. Our entire reality crumbled. Words changed meaning, people looked different, and the world had crushed our future. There was nothing, no feelings, no time, nothing. I was smoking so much marijuana to combat the stress that I went through an ounce a week—that is a lot, believe me—and it wasn't even helping.

A week into this hell, most people would approach me and my kids with despair and sadness and the inevitable "so sorry," which, for the record, doesn't mean shit. Just words about your feeling that we don't have the strength to care about. So there I was, sitting in hell, terrified of each minute headed my way, and what was I going to do with my kids? How was I going to be a father and a puddle of mess at the same time?

At that moment, standing in my front yard, my friend and fellow comedian Jacob Sirof called me to see how I was doing. He was close to my wife, a dear friend. We say hi, and then he says, "You *are* gonna use this widower shit to get some pussy, right?" I exploded into laughter for the first time in a week. My entire life, I never went a week without laughing. Jacob said he was scared to say it, wasn't sure if I would laugh. I told him it was the greatest thing that had happened to me in years. That release was exactly what I needed to think straight. In that moment I knew it would be okay, I could raise these kids alone.

The next few years were still pretty stressful, both kids needed therapy, but we got through it. Stories about my wife were first told with tears but are now told with laughter, like the time I came home from work and Cindy was vacuuming completely nude except for a pair of sexy high heels. "Hi, honey," she said. She cracked me up.

If you can't laugh at it, then it just sucks.[76]

On my tours, people will occasionally describe a terrible event or situation they are dealing with and ask me how they can find the humor in it. I always tell them that I couldn't possibly come up with something they would find amusing without knowing more about them, nor would I want to make light of their personal

---

76 Conor Kellicutt is a San Francisco Bay Area comedian and actor. More of his work can be found at www.conor-comedy.com.

situations. I know that is not the answer they are looking for, but it is an awkward position for me to be put in. As a comedian, I believe that any subject can be a source of humor but I completely recognize that not every person is ready to laugh at any subject. Sometimes it takes time.

I cannot imagine the pain that Conor felt after the death of his wife and I have no idea how I would act if I had to endure a similar tragedy. One thing I am certain of is that, like Conor, I would eventually need a good laugh.

Don't Eat the Poison Berries

It is difficult to think positively all the time. Whether they are bears or unicorns, bad things happen to all of us and negative thoughts are unavoidable. It is perfectly natural to have negative thoughts pop into our head from time to time. In fact, our brain seems to be somewhat disposed to seek out negativity and hold onto it. Psychologists refer to this phenomenon as the "negativity bias."[77] Basically, if we encounter two stimuli, one positive and one negative, our brain is more likely to notice and be affected by the negative stimulus. It sucks, but it's how our brain is wired.

---

77 Roy F. Baumeister et al., "Bad is Stronger than Good," *Review of General Psychology* 5, no. 4 (2001): 323–370.

It makes sense too, if you think about how the brain develops and gathers information about the world it finds itself in. To illustrate this, I like to imagine the challenges that must have been faced by the first human beings, hundreds of thousands of years ago in the savannas of northern Africa. Imagine being one of the first people to explore the area in search of food. Suppose you stumble upon a bush growing some fresh berries that look strangely appealing. You grab a handful, examine them thoroughly, and decide to toss a couple into your mouth. And they are . . . delicious! Sweet and juicy, but not only do they taste great, you suddenly feel energized as the nutrients begin to circulate throughout your body. You just discovered a tasty source of food and it is important for your brain to remember these berries, in case you get hungry in the future.

Now imagine that you encounter a different kind of bush with a different kind of berry. However, this time when you cram a few in your early human mouth they taste terrible. In fact, they make you feel queasy and ill. Maybe one of your buddies, who had a bit more than you, gets sick and dies. The berries, as it turns out, are highly poisonous. Now, although it is extremely important to remember which berries were tasty and nutritious, it is absolutely crucial to your survival to remember the ones that could potentially kill you. It is a simple matter of survival. I often explain the negativity bias this way, with poison berries.

Your brain may require a few encounters with the delicious berries before they are committed to memory, but it will require far fewer experiences to learn about the poison ones. Similarly, think about the act of cooking. It takes a lot of practice to learn how to cook, but you only have to burn yourself once to learn to avoid touching the stove top. It's poison berries. It is adaptive that we learn to identify potential threats as fast as we can, so we naturally favor and pay more attention to negative stimuli than positive stimuli. It makes sense that we are more likely to take notice of, and remember, the bear running toward us than the beautiful sights in the forest.

Obviously, in the modern world very few of us find ourselves in a position where we have to forage for unknown berries for survival. Heck, if I want some berries right now, I can drive to the supermarket down the block and pick up a bag or two. All of them, thankfully, have been preselected and cultivated by human beings who came before me to make sure they are sweet and tasty, or, at the very least, not poisonous. However, our selective preference for negative information influences our thoughts in many other ways.

Romantic relationships offer a great example of this selective preference. Most of us go through a few breakups in our pursuit of that special somebody before we either find them or decide to settle on someone at least moderately tolerable. Relationships are great and can be really healthy, but they are also really stressful and fights happen. Everyone, no matter how awesome they are, has the potential to screw up or even do something intentionally to hurt our feelings. I know that I have screwed up in relationships more than a few times. If you ever find yourself accidentally doing something that hurts your partner, you probably know that from that point forward, that indiscretion seems to be the only thing they remember. They seem to forget all of the thousands of times you were perfectly fine and instead focus on that one time you screwed up. That's poison berries.

Sarah and I first met years ago, when she attended one of my seminars. Recently, we were going through a few storage boxes and came across the notes she took on that day. Curiously, she had written "Poison berries" in her margins and underlined it. To this day we are not sure why, but I do try hard not to piss her off too much.

Another form of pervasive negative thinking is that sometimes we overestimate the likelihood of the worst-case scenario. When I was still a graduate student, I taught classes for the university. One day I asked my students to think of a bad part of town, then I asked them to imagine going there late one night. I asked them to estimate how likely it would be that they would be victimized in some way as a result. I also had them estimate a measure of their level of optimism, and not surprisingly those who were low in optimism estimated a higher probability of being the victim of a crime than those who were more optimistic. What really struck me as interesting was that on average the less optimistic students estimated that they had a 50 percent chance of being victimized if they went to this part of town at night. Here's the thing, I have no idea what the actual crime rates were for this particular area, but I cannot believe they would even have come close to 50 percent. That would imply that half of the people in the neighborhood are being jacked in one way or another every night! We are talking *The Purge* levels of crime here.

Why would they estimate the crime rate to be so high? Well again, the purpose of stress and our bias toward poison berries is to keep us safe. If overestimating the probability of crime, or bear attacks, keeps us away from downtown, or the forest, then that may be unfortunate but at least we get to keep on living.

Sometimes we just overestimate the inconvenience associated with an action.

Before Sarah and I started touring together, I was living in Los Angeles, West Hollywood to be more specific. If you are unfamiliar with the area, West Hollywood is a separate city that is completely surrounded by the city of Los Angeles. In that way, it's a lot like Beverly Hills only with fewer plastic surgeons. West Hollywood, you may be surprised to learn, is located just west of Hollywood. If you have ever driven the Sunset Strip, you were in West Hollywood and I bet you didn't even realize you were in a different city. I loved living there; it is an incredibly vibrant and interesting place, and an extremely liberal community. West Hollywood is also centrally located, which makes it fairly convenient to get around the city by Los Angeles standards.

I moved to Los Angeles for the same reason that a lot of people do: to try and break into film and TV. In the three years I spent there, I didn't get that much screen time (I did manage to get two seconds of my face into a direct-to-DVD piece of garbage movie), but I met a few cool people and learned to network. Occasionally I was invited to entertainment industry events like parties, premieres, or open casting calls. Most of the time they were located in Hollywood or not too far away from home—another advantage of living where I did—but once in a while I was invited to an event in downtown Los Angeles.

Downtown is about ten miles from West Hollywood, which means it takes about four weeks to get there in traffic. Whenever I had an opportunity to attend something downtown, the negative side of my brain would kick in and start actively discouraging me from going. I would think to myself . . .

> *Oh man, all the way downtown? I'll have to leave early enough to deal with traffic. When I get there, it's going to be a pain in the ass to find parking and I will probably have to pay to valet. Plus, do I really know anyone who will be there? Am I really going to meet some movie producer in desperate need of an overweight middle-aged comedian? We are such a rare commodity. I'll spend an hour in traffic, another thirty minutes trying to find parking before I give up and pay the valet just to spend another two hours trying to mingle and schmooze with a bunch of people I'll probably never see again, only to spend another hour driving home in Hollywood-bound traffic. And if I want to go that means I will probably have to put on pants . . .*

Sometimes my overestimation of the inconvenience would prevent me from doing the very thing I was in Los Angeles to do. (And, by the way, downtown Los Angeles has always been one of my favorite places in the city. It has some great historic sites, incredible markets along Broadway, a really cool new arts district, Chinatown, Little Tokyo . . . I'm just saying. I know that most people who visit Los Angeles are interested in seeing Hollywood and spending some time at the beach, but please don't let my stupid anecdote dissuade you from checking out the city's core. You might find some tasty berries, or at least some killer tacos.)

We should not beat ourselves up if we have a hard time being positive (beating ourselves up is the exact opposite of what we should be doing). Our brains are generally more focused on negativity, and even the most positive among us have our moments. However, pervasive negative thinking is ultimately going to interfere with our ability to handle stress, so we should try to do what we can to reduce it before it becomes problematic.

Part of being an optimistic thinker is suppressing negative thoughts. As I previously mentioned, optimistic people have pessimistic thoughts all the time, we just don't dwell on them. One thing that helps is something I have already mentioned: redirecting your train of thought to something else. Literally, anything else. It works for worrying, and it works for all negative thinking in general.

Another thing that I recommend is a practice called "decatastrophization."[78] With this technique, we can use our estimation of the likelihood of the worst-case scenario to help us come to terms with our current situation. I have actually done this, even before I learned that a psychologist had a term for it. When stressed, I would frequently ask myself or others: "What's the worst thing that could happen?" and "What are the chances that will happen?" It is a great way to put things into perspective and reduce negative thinking.

Let me give you an example: imagine once again that you are sitting in traffic and getting frustrated and filled with cortisol. Negative thoughts start creeping in as you get increasingly more stressed. What is the worst-case scenario in traffic? Traffic is usually such a trivial stressor to me that I have a hard time even coming up with a worst-case scenario. I guess, ultimately the worst thing would be that I sit in traffic forever. That I die of starvation

---

78 Albert Ellis, *Reason and Emotion in Psychotherapy* (Oxford, UK: Lyle Stuart, 1962).

sitting in my car, surrounded by a bunch of jack-holes honking their horns. That is probably the worst thing that could happen in traffic, and the likelihood of it happening is extremely low. Besides, I would abandon my car for the nearest sandwich or call to have a pizza delivered to the highway long before it would ever get to that point. I have actually engaged this mental practice in traffic before, and imagining that outcome really does help take the edge off of being a few minutes late for work.

What if the worst thing that could happen has already happened? Well first, that sucks and I am truly sorry that you had to deal with whatever that was. But then, to employ another frequent refrain from my internal dialogue: *It's not the end of the world*. Sometimes the worst thing does happen, but knowing that the worst is behind you means that your situation can only stay the course or improve. It can't get any worse than the worst-case scenario; that is kind of part of the definition. By imagining the worst-case scenario, we put ourselves back in a position to return to optimistic thinking.

To summarize, it is important to understand that we have a natural tendency to focus on negative possibilities and outcomes, and take measures to counter this when it becomes problematic. Changing the course of our train of thought and putting things into perspective can help suppress undesirable negative thoughts.

IN SUMMARY:

- We have a tendency to focus on negativity; we can reduce this by redirecting our thoughts or putting things into perspective.

9

Feeling Overwhelmed
and Exhausted

When I first set out to write this book, I started by thinking not just of the advice and anecdotes that I wanted to share, but of all the common questions people have for me. I also gave my friends an opportunity to submit questions and I have incorporated them throughout. One that I felt deserved its own section came from my friend Jessica. She asked, "What advice would you give for someone who is feeling overwhelmed and exhausted? How does a person turn the downward spiral of stress around and get it moving in the direction of calmness?"

Terrific question, and very relevant. Before I get into it, let me state that in my answer, I am assuming that feeling overwhelmed or exhausted is the result of a short-term or temporary stressful condition, not the result of a longer period of stress slowly wearing someone down and taking its toll on their health. A situation like that may require medical attention and is way beyond the sort of advice I am including here. I am also assuming that the person is not suffering from a nervous breakdown, adrenal failure, or another condition best treated by medicine. Instead I interpret this as what can we do to break the cycle of emotional exhaustion brought on by a normal stress response as it is occurring. People who are dealing with more severe issues can also benefit from this list but should really speak with a physician.

Throughout this book I have given a whole lot of advice, but most of what I have suggested is for developing our ability to manage stress over the long term. The best time to focus on developing our stress-management skills is when we are not currently stressed. You wouldn't wait until the bear was charging you before you picked up this book, right? Unfortunately, people sometimes only seek answers when they need them, not when they are in the best condition to apply those answers. However, when we are feeling pressure and need some immediate relief, there are a few things we can do to help our body calm down.

The first thing, and I know you have heard this one before so please don't stop me, is to breathe. Take a series of deep focused breaths. Yes, you got all the way through this book to read something you already know. *But Brian, breathing is such a simple thing*, you are thinking, *and I am feeling way too overwhelmed for that to do any good!* That's just it, controlling your breathing really does help reduce the effects of stress. Breathing is unlike a lot of bodily functions. It is normally involuntary, meaning that you will breathe regardless of whether you want to or not and often without thinking about it. However, it can be voluntarily controlled. Of all the physiological changes that take place during a stress response, very few of them can be controlled with your conscious mind. You can modify your breathing, but try modifying your blood flow or vasoconstriction (while you are at it, try spelling that correctly without help because I totally just did). As I explained in a previous chapter, when we become stressed, we activate our sympathetic nervous system to get our body ready for action; this includes breathing faster. When we purposely slow down our breathing, it in turn triggers the parasympathetic nervous system to calm us down, and as that system kicks in, the other physiological changes brought on by stress are reduced. Deep breathing is universally recognized as an excellent calming tool, and is a major part of meditation practices. You have heard of it before because it works.

The second thing that I would recommend is exercise. Physical activity, *any* physical activity, is going to help get your body to calm down pretty quickly. This should make perfect sense if you have been paying attention at all throughout this discussion. Stress is the brain's reaction to a perception of threat and it gets the body ready for action, so give it some action. Technically speaking, physical activity is what stress is designed for. All that fighting and fleeing the body is preparing for? Yeah, that's exercise. Exercise is the absolute best way to quickly and effectively reduce stress. I used to have a roommate who struggled with stress management and anger. He had the most amazing coping strategy; whenever he felt a bit agitated he would immediately drop down and bang out a set of push-ups. He'd get back up from the ground, calm and ready to deal with whatever had set him off. You don't have to do push-ups, but if you can squeeze in some sort of intense activity, it is a great way to burn off that cortisol buildup. In fact, consider what happens when you engage your stress response and you do not have a chance for physical activity. For example, imagine you are sitting behind the wheel of a car. You get stressed, your body surges with hormones, and you have nothing to do but sit there and marinate in your own cortisol. Yuck. Exercise is the best way to get immediate relief from stress. It is a shame that so few of us actually do it.

The third thing I will suggest is simply to smile, even if you have to force it. From what I described earlier about the James-Lange Theory of Emotion, you can probably infer that smiling and laughing make us happy. Remember, the brain interprets physio-logical cues from the body to determine its emotional state. There are a few studies that show we can elevate our mood by tricking our brain into thinking it is smiling. One way that works well is to hold a pen, pencil, or similarly shaped object in the mouth side-ways with the teeth.[79] This creates a facial configuration similar to a smile and immediately elevates mood in most people. This is not just a demonstration of the James-Lange theory, but is also my favorite intervention for negative emotion. You can try it yourself: if you are feeling down one day and there's nothing you've done that's made you feel better, put a pen in your mouth! Try it, it can't hurt. Just don't bite down too hard.

There are individual differences of course, but in general, the more we smile, the happier we become. Are you familiar with the phrase "Fake it until you make it"? In this context, it is absolutely

---

79 Fritz Strack, Leonard L. Martin, and Sabine Stepper, "Inhibiting and Facilitating Conditions of the Human Smile: A Nonobtrusive Test of the Facial Feedback Hypothesis," *Journal of Personality and Social Psychology* 54, no. 5 (May 1988): 768–777.

true. Even Botox injections, which inhibit frowning, can increase happiness.[80]

I recommend all three of these interventions on a regular basis, but the one that really seems to resonate with audiences is the pen trick. In fact, after a seminar in Palm Springs, California, I received an awesome email from an attendee who used this trick to cope with the stress of southern California traffic. She wrote:

> The following day I drove into Los Angeles. I had been apprehensive about it, as my husband was staying home (we usually travel together), and although the visit was a positive one, there were a lot of stressors present. Based on your lecture, I concentrated on not worrying and focused on how I was going to have the time to listen to my favorite singer while driving!
>
> I started the drive, traffic was light and Johnny Mathis was singing away. By the time I reached Beaumont, my nerves kicked in. My heart rate was racing, choking sensation, shaky . . . I was having an anxiety attack! Cortisol was coursing through my body! I thought about what you said and, while I didn't have a pen handy, I put my front teeth together and forced myself to smile. And just that one effort immediately stopped the anxiety! The cortisol stopped flowing. I continued to do this off and on for the next twenty miles or so. And for the rest of the trip, if I felt even the slightest hint of anxiousness, I just smiled a big smile and everything was A-OK.

---

80 Michael B. Lewis and Patrick J. Bowler, "Botulinum Toxin Cosmetic Therapy Correlates with a More Positive Mood," *Journal of Cosmetic Dermatology* 8, no. 1 (February 2009): 24–26.

On our next pass through the Palm Springs area, Sarah, Alyssa and I met up with the woman behind the email, Suzanne, and made a new friend.

AND NOW, FOR THE SKIMMERS:

Three things we can do in the moment to calm ourselves down:

- Deep breathing
- Physical exercise
- Force a smile

Money Doesn't Buy Happiness, But Misery Takes Credit

At some point in high school, I had an epiphany. It seemed to me that too many people in the world look back on their high school or college years as the best time of their life while settling down for a less satisfactory adult experience. Maybe I saw too many examples of people with unfulfilled dreams, but whatever it was, I realized that I did not want to peak in high school, or college, or at any point in the past. I wanted to live my life to the fullest at every age and when people asked me about the best time of my life, I would have no problem pointing to the present. I did not want to yearn for the past or point to a possible future. I was not completely off base with this idea; a lot of meditation practices, such as mindfulness, which have been shown to be very helpful in reducing stress, teach people to focus on being present in the moment.

Unfortunately, by the time I got into college, my sensible zen-like realization somehow got warped into something else. Perhaps it was because I was getting closer to taking my position in the workforce, but I started to realize a peculiar paradox. It seemed that money and time were inversely related. As a young college student, I had an abundance of free time but very few resources; however, as a working stiff adult I would be lucky if I had two weeks of vacation time a year but, I imagined, I would have substantially more resources at my disposal. My solution was to experience as much as I could when I had the time to do it, and pay for it later when I had the income. I wish I'd had the wisdom not to live in the moment by sacrificing my future, because in the pursuit of experience I lived way beyond my means. When other college students were living on ramen noodles and cheap beer, I was spending way too much for a guy making his money from burger flipping.

Credit card companies loved consumers like me. They practically passed out preapproved cards at the student union, and I was eager to accept them all. It wasn't long before I had a wallet full of maxed-out credit cards, paying one with another just to keep myself afloat. Eventually, I qualified for student loans, which not only paid my tuition, but gave me enough left over to pay off my higher-interest credit cards. Student loan interest would not accrue until after graduation, so I thought this was a great way to buy myself some time. However, it was the worst financial decision I ever made.

I put myself in major debt to enjoy some extra experiences in college.

You are probably familiar with the phrase "Money can't buy happiness," as it gets tossed around a lot. Whenever I hear it, it is generally used as a morality cue to discourage materialism and greed while reminding people to focus on relationships with other people and other things that truly make them happy. The fact is, research seems to confirm that money does not buy happiness for most people. Incremental changes in income do not correlate with incremental changes in happiness.[81] However, as one wealthy golfer said to another in a well-known *New Yorker* cartoon by Pat Byrnes, "Researchers say I'm not happier for being richer, but do you know how much researchers make?"

I qualified my previous statement by saying "most people" because research does show that one particular group of people does report greater levels of happiness when they receive more money: those who live below the poverty line. When you are broke, then yes, mo' money equals mo' happy. Simply put, money makes poor people happier because it helps to relieve the stress of poverty. When you are concerned about basic needs like food, shelter, and safety, it is hard to be happy all the time. Those are some very real bears about to attack. Recent research seems to suggest that the bar for happiness may be higher than just getting

---

81 There are lots of examples, but one poll that I often refer to is the *Time* magazine/SRBI Poll (2004).

above the poverty line, but I suspect that is because of the debt ratio. When debt is high, even a high income is not enough to alleviate the stress of basic needs. This is why you find people living in cities like San Francisco, earning a reasonably high salary and barely keeping their head above water (I know from experience). However, once we remove the stress of poverty or debt, additional income does not bring about additional happiness.

This is counterintuitive to a lot of us because we have firsthand experience that a little more money brings joy. Early in my career, I remember every tiny increase in my hourly wage, which started at $3.35 an hour because I am that old, as putting a huge smile on my face, and my first salaried position after graduate school had me dancing in the streets. Those experiences are enough to train our brain into thinking that lasting happiness has a price tag and someday when we hit it big in Vegas (or the lottery), everything will be awesome. However, the happiness we feel when we get a nice shot of cash is a fleeting, momentary happiness. Eventually, we get used to it and need more to feel momentarily happy again. Psychologists refer to this as the "hedonic treadmill," or "hedonic adaptation."[82]

I like to explain hedonic adaption by looking back on the cars I have owned throughout my life. I remember when I was still a poor high school student trying really hard not to peak. I remember having to walk five miles uphill to school, both ways, sometimes knee-deep in thick central Texas snow; also I had no feet. We couldn't afford feet until I was a junior, so I had to compete in the jalapeño-eating contest on stumps. Like a lot of kids,

---

82 Daniel Kahneman, Edward Diener, and Norbert Schwarz, eds., *Well-Being: Foundations of Hedonic Psychology* (New York, NY: Russell Sage Foundation, 1999).

especially those in rural Texas, I could barely wait to get my driver's license. It was going to make me so happy, and eventually it did. I worked hard for it, excelled in my driving classes, aced my exam, and even got a fresh haircut to have my picture taken. Having my driver's license made me so happy that for at least a week I stared at it all the time, even slept with it under my pillow. My mother occasionally let me drive her car and I was thrilled for the opportunity, but eventually I got used to it and adapted. My license was no longer a source of joy, so I started setting my sights on buying my own car. I knew that having my own set of wheels would finally make me happy and saved up until I could purchase my first car. That car, pardon my French, was a total piece of shit. But I loved it. I washed it and drove it as often as I could and parked it outside my bedroom window so I could keep an eye on it. Eventually, I adapted. Simply owning a car no longer provided me with any joy. I needed a nicer car, a bigger car, a car to impress with, a car with modern technology . . . maybe a Mustang convertible . . . after all, roofs are for suckers. Truthfully, I have never really cared all that much about cars, but you can see how that sort of behavior may land someone on a treadmill of sorts, and deep in debt if they are not careful.

I recently had a conversation with a friend who asked me if he should go to a concert. My friend has been struggling financially the entire time that I have known him, and has endured brief periods of homelessness when he was forced to live out of his car. I recommended that he save the money, and he replied: "It's only ten bucks, what is the point of saving it if I will still be broke?" I completely understand the mentality, as I used to share it, but it is an attitude that keeps us broke. Imagine a dieter who says, "It's only an extra slice of cake, what is the point if I will still be fat?" Or "What are five sit-ups going to do for me? I might as well just enjoy sitting on the couch." Unfortunately, those thoughts may ring true, but eventually if we want to change our situation, we have to break the behavioral cycle that keeps us there. Those small steps eventually add up.

It is true that money does not buy lasting happiness, but living with money in the bank and with minimal debt is a great way to reduce stress. Without all that pesky stress getting in the way, you are free to pursue the things that actually bring about happiness. You know, like some of the things I discussed in previous sections.

One of the biggest single sources of stress in our lives is money and how we convince other people to give it to us through work. I mentioned previously the importance of feeling in control. Unless you are your own boss, work is usually a situation in which you have very little control. Having some money in the bank is a great way to increase that sense of control. Think about it, feeling in control means you feel like you have the ability to either solve the problem or remove yourself from it whenever you want. Having money in the bank may not suddenly make your boss tolerable or help you solve your situation at work, but you know that as bad as that situation gets, you have the means to leave whenever you want. That is a sense of control, and a powerful means to reduce the impact that a shitty job can have on your health. People who live paycheck to paycheck don't have the same sense of control.

Being surrounded by creative types, I frequently hear people say things like "I don't care about money." I understand what they mean, that their primary interest is something other than trying to accumulate wealth, but being broke is a source of stress and stress contributes to a whole lot of ill health. I wish they cared just a little more about money.

Eventually I was able to pay off all of my college debt and set a little savings aside. It took a lot of sacrifice, and a great deal of commitment through the years, but a whole bunch of little steps added up. (Now if only I could tackle those extra slices of cake.) I now live life a bit closer to the epiphany I had in high school, and I can honestly say that every year since I have been debt-free has been the best year of my life, each one better than the one before it. Even my willingness to start a family was related to my changing financial situation.

AND NOW, FOR THE SKIMMERS:

- Money, and related issues, are some of the biggest sources of stress. Saving and living with minimal debt can be a tremendous help to alleviating stress.

I was able to successfully pull myself out of the pit of a tough financial situation, but I am by no means an expert on the subject. What worked for me worked because of my unique set of circumstances, and probably would not work for a lot of other people. I am an example, not an expert. Who do you think would give you better advice on how to lose weight, the person who has devoted their life to researching weight loss or the person who has personally managed to lose one hundred pounds? Of course the expert is going to provide us with advice that is more likely to be applicable to our lives, but that doesn't stop the examples from writing books. Trusting an example rather than an expert is a common fallacy, and if you need sound financial advice, I will always defer to an expert.

But I can offer a couple of bits of advice that helped me. The first was to realize that to achieve my goal, there were simply some things I would have to do without. A lot of things, actually. I cut out spendy habits like dining out, and shopping as a recreational activity. I also sacrificed certain luxuries like cable TV and internet. Cutting cable eventually led to less TV consumption, and without home internet, I spent more time on other activities. If I needed to check something online, I used free Wi-Fi somewhere or waited until I went to work the next day. It was also an easier time to live without a cell phone. After that, I started looking at all sorts of ways to spend less, tracking and scrutinizing my bank statements each week.

Second, I had to tear away the debt. Each month, a way-too-large chunk of my income went to make minimum payments on a few credit cards and a student loan. I decided to start paying them off in the order of their balance, so after making my minimum payments, I sent as much extra money to my lowest-balance card as possible. With online banking this was a snap, and I got to save money on stamps and envelopes. Some months, I would send three to five payments to the same creditor, slowly chipping away at the balance. With each debt I eliminated, there was one less monthly payment to make and more money available to chip away at the next one.

Third, I had to increase my income as much as possible. With my full-time position, I was unable to take on a part-time job or commit to any other work, so that was a limitation. However, I found I could generate income by selling off unneeded posessions. I sold appliances, furniture, collectibles, and anything else I could spare on eBay, and I sold books on Amazon. In the process, I discovered that one of my books was rare and it brought in a nice profit. I searched eBay for the same book, bought several copies there for much less than my copy sold for, and I flipped them on Amazon for another nice profit. I also took in a roommate for extra income and to reduce expenses. If Airbnb, Uber, or Lyft had existed then, I definitely would have jumped on those opportunities as well.

Through a combination of reducing consumption, commiting to paying off my debts, and increasing my income however I could, I was able to change my situation. Come to think of it, that's not all that specific to me, but you should still consult with an expert.

The Biggest Irony of My Modern Life

Did you know it is possible to suffer the effects of stress without actually being aware of the stress itself? Sometimes we can't locate the source of the tension—no attacking bears, no motionless traffic, not even any imaginary unicorns to be found—and yet, somehow, we experience a full-on activation of our stress response.

Having a family makes people healthy—the statistical evidence says as much. On average, married men live longer than single men and people with children live longer than people without. Partners care about our well-being and encourage us to make healthier choices, and children keep us physically active in a time in our life where we have a tendency to be sedentary. Knowing this, I somehow avoided both for the majority of my life and managed to survive as a childless, single man into my forties.

Not that I was ever a model of good health—I could be a great "before" photo—but I managed to get by without developing any significant complications. I have been overweight my entire life, but I have not yet experienced any of the negative health effects of carrying excess body weight. Except, of course, the bane of every fat person's existence: stairs. It all comes down to poor lifestyle choices regarding diet and exercise. Choices that I have been unconsciously making, yet consciously aware of (like sitting on the couch instead of hitting the gym or absent-mindedly ordering chocolate cookies). However, I know that my stress management contributes to my health, and I know that it is possible to offset bad lifestyle choices by managing stress well. The health risks associated with obesity include hypertension and diabetes, whereas the health risks associated with prolonged stress include—guess what—hypertension and diabetes. Imagine being overweight *and* metaphorically carrying the weight of the world in stress. I may have had bad eating and exercise habits, but at least I wasn't stressed.

Then came Sarah, whom I won't disparage, and then came a baby in a baby carriage—or however the old playground song goes.

Sarah is an occupational therapist and as such is a part of the healthcare community. I sometimes work with people in healthcare, but I am really just a guy with a degree in psychology who tells jokes. There is a cliché that when a woman finds a man, she wants to change him, and I was a big potential occupational therapy project. There is another cliché that men are very reluctant to seek healthcare, and yeah, that was me. I didn't even get health insurance until President Obama forced me to. I guess that despite our unconventional lifestyle, Sarah and I are just a couple of clichés.

"You need to see a doctor!" she would say. But I didn't want to see a doctor; I knew I needed to lose weight and stubbornly thought that was all I would learn from paying to see a professional. The tipping point came when we learned that our daughter was going to join our lives. Even then, Sarah had to convince me to go in for a checkup. During some time off of our touring, we went to stay with my parents and I scheduled what I thought was going to be a very routine appointment at an urgent care clinic.

My blood pressure was high. Scary high. Like I could die any minute high.

For the first time in my life I feared that my poor life choices had finally caught up with me, and just before the birth of my daughter. I was scared and started to stress. I was already going to be older than most first-time fathers, but I hated to think about having my time with Alyssa cut short because of a heart attack or stroke. Besides, my brain is all I have! I spent my entire life trying to fill it: from Shakespeare to the Talmud, the formulas of Einstein, and Beatles songs, even paraphrasing this quote from the 1980 movie *Flash Gordon*.[83] Actually, it probably holds a lot more movie quotes than literature and I have never even read the Talmud, but still. Nobody lives forever, but I didn't want to miss out on spending time with my daughter if I could do something about it.

In my consultation with the doctor I mentioned some other issues that I hadn't really thought much about until then but that were probably related. For the previous several years I had been experiencing body pain, aches in my muscles and joints. I had been increasingly lethargic and prone to uncontrollable, almost narcoleptic, bouts of sleep. All of this I had dismissed as being an effect of my weight, which had been steadily increasing over roughly the same time period despite a relatively healthy diet and exercise. The doctor turned to Sarah and asked, "Does he snore?" Like a grizzly bear in winter he snores.

The doctor immediately pegged me as someone with sleep apnea and expressed his concern.

I had actually suspected that I had sleep apnea for a long time at that point, at least a couple of years. I had taken a comedian friend on tour with me for a few weeks and I remember that on every drive between gigs he would fall dead asleep riding shotgun after downing multiple bottles of 5-hour Energy. I would drive and he would snore, making him one of the least interesting travel companions ever. Every so often his breathing would stop and he would wake up briefly to utter something incomprehensible before falling back asleep to continue the cycle (much like his

---

83 As a true eighties child, I am paraphrasing Dr. Hans Zarkov's explanation of why Ming's memory-wipe device did not work on him: "As I was going under, I started to recite Shakespeare, the Talmud, the formulas of Einstein, anything I could remember, even a song from the Beatles."

act). He and I were about the same size physically and I knew that I had a strong snore, but until I saw him struggle in his sleep, I never made the connection that I might be having the same issue. I certainly never thought that I needed to treat it. Actually, I figured I would lose weight, as my weight tends to go up and down, and that would take care of the problem for me.[84] Besides, I thought it was nothing more serious than extreme snoring. And the girls can always buy earplugs.

What can I say? I am not a medical doctor.

After that consultation I decided to do a little research. I learned that sleep apnea is more than extreme snoring. Periodically throughout the night, my throat would block the passage of air to my lungs. As is completely understandable, not being able to receive oxygen is identified as a major threat by the brain. Just like any other stressor, only potentially more serious, this blockage causes the body to freak out and panic. In response, the body produces a massive dose of cortisol to wake me up. This happened about three or four times a night, making it virtually impossible to get a good night's sleep and causing me to be lethargic and sleepy during the day.

As soon as I learned about the cortisol connection, everything suddenly made sense to me. Not only was I receiving periodic jolts of cortisol throughout the night, but sleep deprivation itself is interpreted by the body as a form of stress (our bodies kind of need to sleep). Therefore, the body reacts to it physiologically just as it does any other form of stress.[85] Cortisol, the stress hormone,

---

84 That's not true by the way, there are a lot of fit people who suffer from sleep apnea as well.

85 G. Takada et al., "Sleep Apnea and its Association with the Stress System, Inflammation, Insulin Resistance and Visceral Obesity," *Sleep Medicine Clinics* 2, no. 2 (June 2007): 251–261.

is a major factor in heart disease, obesity, diabetes, impotence, and pretty much any mental illness you can think of. For who knows how many years, without realizing it, I had been jacking up my cortisol levels overnight, and probably every day I was sleep deprived. As I previously discussed, our stress response is not intended to be activated for a long term and this was contributing to my blood pressure, my bodily aches and pains, and probably a bunch of other symptoms I neglected to list. Sleep apnea was also making it extremely difficult to achieve my other goals during the day (like staying awake), and was almost certainly a factor in my difficulty with managing my weight.

I learned that people die of sleep apnea and apnea-related illnesses. A lot of people. Thankfully there is a treatment for the disease; it involves a machine that provides continuous positive airway pressure (CPAP) to prevent the throat from closing during sleep. There are other treatments, but for me the nasal CPAP was enough. Other than feeling like my nostrils had been deflowered, my first night wearing it was the best night of sleep I had ever had. My body was so used to being tired all the time that being sleep deprived had become my normal state. After my second night with my CPAP, I woke up feeling better than I had felt in a very long time. I felt incredibly alert and energetic. Not that I was ready to go for a jog or anything, but my body didn't ache when we walked around the neighborhood and I didn't find myself falling asleep at my computer or needing naps. I felt better in ways I didn't even know were possible.

The thing about sleep apnea is that you spend a lot less time in restorative deep sleep because you keep being interrupted and have to start over every time your brain falls back asleep. Sleep is divided into five stages based on brain activity, labeled 1 through 4, and REM for the rapid eye movements that occur at that stage. In an uninterrupted sleep cycle, we start to doze off with stage 1, become less aware and more relaxed with stages 2 and 3, and enter deep sleep with stage 4. With apnea, our brain may be awakened before it ever gets to stage 4 and beyond. This is a major concern because slow-wave sleep, and REM, are the restorative stages when the body grows (if it has growing to do), makes repairs to and strengthens muscles, and solidifies memories of the things we've learned or experienced during the day. An absence of slow-wave sleep means we aren't growing or benefiting much from exercise and are probably having difficulty learning and remembering. Dreaming usually occurs in REM sleep, and a side effect of sleep apnea is not dreaming. Along with feeling tired and wanting to fall asleep at inappropriate times, my brain often went directly into REM. I would doze off and be dreaming while on my lunch break, or sitting at my computer trying to get work done, or in probably one of the worst situations imaginable, sitting at a red light in traffic.

On my first day of CPAP treatment, according to my charts, my brain spent significantly longer time in REM than it usually does, as if it was trying to make up for lost time. After my first week on the machine, I was not only sleeping better, but dreaming again.

Another thing about sleep apnea is that it contributes to the development of bad sleep habits, and therefore perpetuates a pretty bad downward spiral. For as long as I can remember, I had always had trouble falling asleep at night and waking up in the morning. This schedule is pretty typical for a comedian, but it does make it hard to graduate high school, and oversleeping introduces its own stress. I even worried about oversleeping. Over time my sleeping habits got worse and worse until I got to a point where I could not fall asleep unless my body was ready to completely knock itself out. I would lie in bed, my mind racing, in a futile attempt to catch some Zs. Most nights when I was younger I watched television, or as an adult I surfed the internet, until my body could not take it anymore and I crashed.

My mornings were equally difficult, often with three or four alarms set to go off that I repeatedly hit snooze to stop, or slept through through entirely. On a few occasions when I had an important reason to wake up early the next day, I purposely slept with the lights on in my room. This may seem counterintuitive; the lights would make it harder to fall asleep, but they also made it easier to wake up. Typically, regardless of how much sleep I got the night before, I would wake up groggy, feel unrefreshed, and take way too long to start my day. As a bonus, my sleep/wake habits completely annoyed anyone sharing a bed or room with me. And, in at least one situation, my neighbors. One day while working at my first job after graduate school, I came home to my apartment building to find a note on my door complaining about my morning alarm ritual.

Three weeks into my CPAP treatment I could already see a major change in my sleeping habits. I went to bed every night at a decent hour (decent for me, usually around eleven) and woke up early every morning without the use of an alarm. I couldn't believe how early I was getting up, and how completely refreshed I was feeling every day. To this day, I still wake up without an alarm clock, which is something I couldn't imagine doing when I was younger.

After my diagnosis, I wrote about sleep apnea on my social media accounts, hoping to raise awareness. People asked me if the mask was uncomfortable and told me that they had a hard time using theirs consistently. It did take some getting used to, but the slight discomfort of nose violation is nothing compared to the pain of not sleeping properly night after night—or the potential health issues associated with apnea, as well as the risks and the other side effects. Perhaps more guys would use their CPAP machine if the mask was shaped like Darth Vader's or Iron Man's. Or maybe they would be more likely to wear their masks if they knew that total badass Airborne paratroopers also wear them. Yup, my buddy Cuban from the interview earlier uses one right before he jumps out of a *friggin' airplane* and then eats a bowl of nails and broken glass for breakfast.[86]

After using my CPAP for nearly six months, I noticed a few long-term effects and positive changes to my life. For example, my weight loss. I would never claim that sleep apnea was the only contributor to my lifelong struggle with obesity; childhood laziness was probably a big factor as well. I didn't get fat because of sleep apnea, but having it very likely contributed, with a lifetime of lower energy and heightened cortisol levels. Conversely, as I gained

---

86 Please, he does not do this to my knowledge.

weight my apnea symptoms got progressively worse, to the point that I was gaining weight despite maintaining a relatively healthy diet. It was truly a downward spiral. Thankfully, after six months of treatment, I lost nearly forty pounds, which is awesome not just because I dropped a few sizes and my modeling career picked up (yeah, right), but because the weight loss also reduced my apnea symptoms. To paraphrase my financial advisor, who also suffers from sleep apnea, it may be possible to lose enough excess weight that the machine won't be necessary. Trust me, upward spirals feel so much better.

After almost a year of treatment, Sarah and I returned to Montreal for a visit to check on our condo and enjoy another summer in Quebec. The city of Montreal takes its name from a mispronunciation of the towering Mount Royal that sits smack in the middle of the island. Like Twin Peaks in San Francisco, the mountain is mostly parkland and affords some of the most spectacular views of the city. The jewel in the crown is a beautiful chalet that is located just a short, slightly uphill, 1,196-meter walk (about three-quarters of a mile) from the closest parking lot. It is an easy hike and every year thousands of visitors come to soak in the absolutely breathtaking view it offers of downtown. The first time I attempted that moderate hike was before starting with the CPAP and I was probably in the worst physical condition of my life. That short hike kicked my ass. It is crazy to think about, but just walking a couple of blocks of distance caused me incredible back pain and I needed to stop and rest several times. My knees ached as I walked, my sides hurt so bad that I had to stop and rest several times, and I lost my breath, all while hundreds of people in all shapes and sizes whizzed by me as if I was standing still. On this latest visit, we decided to walk out to the chalet again and I felt none of that. Soon, Alyssa will be running around and I'll be ready for her (well, maybe not as ready as I'd like to be).

I have always been concerned about managing stress and happiness, and I have always led a happy, stress-free life. Occasionally, I am haunted by memories of events when I did not have energy to do things. I missed opportunities, fell asleep during concerts, movies, and other performances (seriously, I once missed half of a Cirque du Soleil show and those tickets weren't cheap), and disappointed people around me. I can only imagine that the way I feel about some things is similar to how a recovering addict might feel about some of their past behavior. But rather than ruminate on the past, I appreciate the present and look forward to continued improvement.

Clarity of mind and more energy. Who would have thought that having your heart jump-start your breathing several times a night could be so bad for you? Now, I breathe better during the day; I rarely cough or clear my throat, and I don't snore at night. I am a better public speaker, I have more focus, and I seem to be a better writer, although I will let you be the judge of that. However, way more importantly, I am a better partner to Sarah, and I am a better father to Alyssa.

I always knew that having children would make me healthier, I just did not anticipate that becoming a father would help my life in this way. I figured Alyssa would get me running to chase after her and increase my physical activity through games and sports, but even before she was born my daughter was having a positive impact on my life. I was already highly resilient, positive, and optimistic, but my daughter has made me healthier. I hope that when she is older she can look back on her life and say the same about her dad. Whoever he is.

10

———

Facing Challenges

From about the time I started planning this book to when I sat down in Denver to begin writing, many people who follow me on social media began sending me articles about a baby named Harper Yeats. Harper was less than six months old and had already traveled to all fifty states in the US.[87] That's a remarkable feat that most adults will probably not accomplish; it is understandable that she received a bit of attention from news networks while on her journey with her parents. The reason why so many people thought to share this story with me is that earlier in the year, my daughter, Alyssa, accomplished the same thing at the age of one. It hadn't occurred to either Sarah or myself that our baby had set some sort of record, but a little research

———

87 To learn more about her story, see Faith Karimi, "Harper Yeats Will Have Traveled to All 50 States This Week. She's Only 5 Months Old," *CNN*, October 15, 2018, https://www.cnn.com/travel/article/harper-yeats-50-states-record-trnd/index.html.

indicated that the youngest known person to travel to all fifty states did so by the age of three. Shortly after I found that out, Harper came along and set a new record for baby travel. So much for the glory, but at least *we* know that for a brief few months Alyssa held the title.

As with Harper's parents, Sarah and I did not plan on taking our daughter on such a journey, it just worked out that way. With my speaking engagements and other events, and Sarah's occupational therapy contracts, our existing tour schedule took us to forty-five states. When we realized this, we decided to add the remaining five so our daughter could have bragging rights. Thankfully, three of them, Wisconsin, North Dakota, and South Dakota, were all within an easy driving distance of Minneapolis, Minnesota, where I had a couple of remaining gigs, and we found a great deal on flights from there to Alaska and Hawaii, the other two. With some last-minute planning, Alyssa got to visit all fifty states and even celebrated her first birthday on beautiful Waikiki Beach. In between, she also made it to five provinces in Canada. Obviously, she will not remember much from her adventures, but that may work in our favor as it would be incredibly difficult and expensive to keep coming up with better birthday experiences.

Before I get too deep into this section, you should know that I am not going to end it by recommending that you take a baby on a whirlwind road trip to relieve stress. That would be ridiculous and probably fairly difficult for most people, although making the baby in preparation would be a lot of fun. I don't even think Sarah and I would repeat the journey unless our circumstances required so. If we ever have another child, um . . . sorry, kid. You should have been born first.

My reason for sharing this story with you is to offer a different sort of advice to parents. When we first announced that Sarah was pregnant, so many of our friends asked us if we were going to settle down somewhere. We did not, and we had no plans to, but we found it interesting how so many people assumed that we would. Not only is traveling directly related to our livelihood, but we really enjoy the lifestyle. Then there were other peculiar questions or comments we received from other parents, like the couple who had not been out to a restaurant in a year because of their baby or the friend that claimed she hadn't been out past eight o'clock. We soon realized how many people out there seemed to think childbirth was like hitting a giant pause button on adult life. It is not, and it certainly does not have to be.

Figuring out how to incorporate children into activities requires a whole lot of problem-solving, which I hear is good for the brain. There are plenty of books and other resources out there that are full of tips on how to parent, and both psychology and occupational therapy degrees offer some insight, but really you cannot anticipate or prepare in advance for all the challenges. For example, three weeks after she was born, our daughter flew on her first airplane (ironically to Minneapolis; if only we'd had the foresight to visit the neighboring states then). Sarah and I did a little research and gave ourselves plenty of extra time and it was still a mess. Mainly, we hadn't appreciated how cumbersome the additional stroller and car seat would be after parking our car. By our next flight out, this one to Washington, we had a new plan: we would unload everything curbside at the terminal where Sarah and Alyssa waited while I returned the rental car. By the third flight, we had a system of checking everything but the stroller curbside, then using the stroller to navigate the airport before checking it at the terminal. In two months and only three flights, we went from novice traveling parents to experts. In the process, Alyssa made it to her first sixteen states.

Flying presented opportunities to problem-solve, but our first cross-country road trip was a definite learning experience. Usually the cities we tour are only a couple of hours apart, but we had an unusual situation when I was scheduled to speak at Rutgers University in New Jersey and again exactly one week later in Newport, Oregon, which, if I remember this correctly, is nowhere near New Jersey. To put even more strain on our travel, I scheduled a book signing in Pittsburgh, Pennsylvania, in between these speaking gigs. This gave us five days to drive over twenty-six hundred miles, which seemed really doable when I booked these gigs as a hardworking, hard-partying father of none. As we soon learned, two-month-old babies do not have a high tolerance for long drives. However, we adapted. Sarah invented an activity we called "truck stop tummy time" and on our third day, I noticed that we seemed to be stopping for diaper changes way too frequently. Because I am a research scientist at heart, I started keeping track of our "miles per diaper" and found that we were averaging about twenty-seven miles per Huggie. We were going through diapers faster than normal and at the rate we were stopping to change them, we were not going to make it to Oregon in time. Then it occurred to us that Alyssa's brain may have learned that every time she let one go, we pulled over and Mommy would pull her out of the car seat. She got changed, but she also got company, which was probably more important to her. Her behavior was receiving both negative reinforcement (removing the soiled diaper) and positive reinforcement (Mommy time), and with two opportunities for reinforcement at once, she increased the frequency of making us stop. To test this hypothesis, we rearranged the car so that Sarah could ride in the back with the baby and our miles per diaper went back up to previous levels. As we rolled into Newport with time to spare, I wondered if my diaper miles data was something I could publish. Turns out, I could.

Look, our experiences may not be typical, but the point I hope you take away from all of this is that although having a child forces you to make some adjustments, it should not prevent you from living a full life. For us, that full life includes traveling and public appearances; for someone else it could mean maintaining their social life or continuing to pursue their hobbies. For a moment, consider the alternative. Imagine what effect becoming a new parent would have on someone who, instead of stepping up to the challenges, chooses to reduce their activity, withdraw socially, and spend all of their time with a screaming newborn. I can't say for sure, but I don't think anyone would be in their happiest state under those circumstances. It is no wonder that so many of my early seminar attendees assumed that I was unstressed because I did not have a family.

I have mentioned the importance of maintaining good problem-solving skills. Well, a lot of life is about challenges and whether or not we successfully overcome them. Sometimes to stay physically and mentally healthy in the modern world, we need to challenge ourselves so that when life hits us, we are ready. Parenthood presents certain challenges, or problems, and like any problem, solving them increases resilience. Not solving them, you know . . . doesn't.

For more than three years, Sarah and I have been living a nomadic lifestyle. We love it and plan to continue doing so as long as it makes sense for us, but it is not a lifestyle I would recommend to anyone. Not that I would discourage anyone considering it, but for most people it probably would not make much sense. Besides, it is not like we spend all our time relaxing at beach resorts and sipping margaritas (actually, we never do that). However, I do recommend travel in general. Traveling outside of the comfort zone of home brings a lot of opportunities to problem solve (although hopefully you won't find yourself in a situation like my brother did in Mexico), even if it is just a short vacation.

I have read articles and seen plenty of videos passed around the internet that imply that some large portion of Americans, maybe half, fail to use their annual vacation benefit from their job. Take your damn vacation! Go somewhere awesome and do something new and different. What I think is really healthy about vacation isn't the sightseeing or partying, it is the mind-set that it puts you in. When you are on vacation, you become willing to try things you have never done before and are much more open to new experiences. Never been scuba diving or eaten at a Brazilian barbeque? Well, when in Rome! Rome is in Brazil, right? Also, because our vacation time is limited there is a sense of urgency to our activities. You only have so much time off before going back to your regular boring life, so get out there and take a selfie in front of the Grand Canyon. It's now or never, Judy.

The first time I visited Hawaii, it was for a two-week vacation. During that time, I saw about thirteen Hawaiian sunsets. I usually don't make an effort to take in the sunset, it sets every day regardless of where I am. But for some reason I felt compelled to watch the sun go down over the ocean in Hawaii as often as I could. Why? Because I only had so many opportunities to do so before I left. The vacation mind-set helps create an urgency to take advantage of opportunities for joy.

Challenging our mind with new experiences keeps us healthy. Vacations, and the mind-set they inspire, help deal with burnout. So take them. You don't have to go somewhere exotic (you know, like Denver), in fact, you may not even have to leave your town. Just leave your comfort zone. When I worked in the corporate world, I valued my paid time off more than other benefits, and I made sure that I used it. But I also considered any day that I was not in the office as a vacation day, as unpaid time off. I try to encourage people to adopt the vacation mind-set even when exploring their own city. Visit that market downtown or check out a park. Every city has something to offer, and too frequently we take these opportunities for granted. There is no urgency when we think we can do it any time, so we never do it. I know well-traveled people who live in San Francisco and have been to Europe but have never been to Alcatraz. I know Chicagoans who have never been to the Art Institute. I know people in Minneapolis who have never seen the St. Paul winter ice castles. And there are people in Oklahoma who have never read a book.[88]

---

88 I'm just saying, there is a reason the song is not "Sweet Home Oklahoma."

Carving a Carousel

Living in Denver puts Sarah and me in close proximity to one of our favorite places in the world, the Carousel of Happiness in Nederland, Colorado. Sarah first stumbled onto it a few years ago on a drive through the Rocky Mountains, and took me there on one of our first dates. We have since visited with Alyssa a few times, whenever our travels took us through this area, and now we feel fortunate to be so close.

At almost three thousand feet above the Mile High City, Nederland is a quaint town up in the mountains, and a beautiful place to visit. It is only a short drive up from Boulder, and the drive alone makes it worth going as coming in from any direction provides breathtaking views. It is a small town, and one of the central points of interest is the carousel, which is very easy to find. Maybe some tourists might pass up a carousel ride, especially adults traveling without children, but discovering gems like this is one of the reasons Sarah and I love to travel. This is not an ordinary carousel; this is a ride with a story.

During the Vietnam War, as our soldiers were subjected to unimaginable stress, a young marine named Scott Harrison frequently found comfort in a tiny music box his sister had mailed him. Holding it to his ear, the music helped remind him of the world outside of his horrific circumstances. According to the

Denver Post, it helped him survive.[89] He said, "One wants to go to a simpler, quieter place in one's head, and I was having dreams of carousels." When he returned home, he started to give life to that dream and in 1986 acquired the frame of an old carousel from Utah. For the next twenty-six years he worked to restore it by hand-carving all of the animals. A project born of a unique strategy to cope with incredible stress, he very fittingly named it the Carousel of Happiness, and happiness is something that it inspires in everyone who visits.

To date, Alyssa has sat on three of his hand-carved animals, and I can attest to the joy and excitement that the carousel brings her. And her parents.

As luck would have it, I was able to speak with Scott about his work and the happiness it inspires.

BK: In your own words, how would you describe the Carousel of Happiness?

Scott: I would just describe it as . . . a kind of magical place where people come in, and like any carousel, it's a fun thing. You don't go anywhere, you just kind of go around in circles. But we don't charge much; we charge one dollar a ride and we just do it for fun. It's just turned out to be much better than what I had thought. It was a selfish project at first, it was something I thought about for a while, and something that seemed like I could do. And then it just turned out to be something that took off on its own, and we have weddings, and memorial services, and lots of big groups

---

89 Julie Hoffman Marshall, "Vet Has a Passion for Merrymaking, *Denver Post*, last updated May 7, 2016, https://www.denverpost.com/2008/08/28/vet-has-a-passion-for-merrymaking/.

come. We have more adults that ride than kids. It's been a little bit of a healing place for a lot of people to come and just sit and get out of their heads, and enjoy the atmosphere watching people ride if they don't ride.

BK: I can see it as a healing place. It feels very therapeutic. How did you get started on it?

Scott: I just started carving.... this was in '85 or '86. After I got out of Vietnam in '68, I carved a couple of animals. I saw an exhibit of one hundred-year-old carousel animals, and there was this one rabbit that had a wise-looking expression and face, and I wanted to replicate that, to see if I could give a wooden animal some sort of substance. So the first animal I did was a rabbit, and I didn't get exactly what I had seen, but I felt like I could keep working at it and I was enjoying the carving.

BK: So would you say that the carving process was therapeutic in itself?

[Scott explained that in the time between the war and his arrival in Nederland, he began working with Amnesty International and created an Urgent Action Network to campaign against torture. The work, although rewarding, did come with stress.]

Scott: When we moved here, we had a one-year-old and a four-year-old. We didn't have a TV at the time, so when we put them to bed, I would just go out to the shop and carve. And frankly that pattern of my life just kept going like that for a couple of decades here in Nederland. Worked in the office, and then I'd go out and carve one animal at a time—and it helped me deal with the stress. Frankly, I thought I was past the combat part of Vietnam, and was just using the other side of my brain for that. I wouldn't say artistic, I would say it's the inconsequential part of my life where nobody, at the time, nobody was waiting for a carousel to be built. I was just doing it for my own peace of mind. It wasn't on deadlines like my work was. And the animals are whimsical and a little silly. That's how I dealt with, I guess one would say, the stress of that subject matter of torture.

BK: And out of that came this place of healing. Can you tell me about some of the experiences you have witnessed at the carousel?

Scott: This is unexpected because I was in my own head in trying to create this carousel. I was just building the pieces of it one at a time, and I've got to say, I wasn't smart enough to try to see the effect it would have on people. But if you are there for more than an hour, you'll see people cry out of either joy or just pure emotion.

We have a lot of older people come in buses from senior centers and stuff. And they're emotional because they think of their past and the carousel in their past.

Others just come and get emotional about the, maybe the simplicity of it, the disengagement that you're offered by getting on an animal and going around in a circle. I don't know quite, or haven't figured all that out, but there have been some times [I've seen it happen]. I'll tell you one time, a couple years ago, a local TV station did a piece on it. I wasn't there for most of it. I went in and just did a short little interview with the reporter. He stayed most of the day with his camera crew. And while he was there, he noticed this woman who was on oxygen. A middle-aged woman sitting on one of the window seats and watching people go around. She wasn't riding it. And he noticed her and he went over and talked to her. And it turned she was in stage 4 breast cancer, terminal. And she would come up on the bus from Boulder just to get out of her head, you know? Get away from her own situation. That was actually several years ago and it spoke to me about how, you know, for a lot of different reasons, it can be a help for people who find . . . I don't know what to say that doesn't sound cliché . . . kind of find a happy place.

BK: Well, it is the Carousel of Happiness. That said, is there anything else on the horizon?

Scott: Well about four years ago, I started another project. Using the same kind of similar components of what the Carousel of Happiness is. This is creating a healing space for people to go. People who have had trauma in their lives. At the time I was working with people with PTSD and since then I've been thinking, you know, we all need some quiet space and quiet time in our lives. So it's really for everybody but I've designed it for people who have had trauma in their lives.

I wanted to create a quiet space but still use wooden animals with their sympathetic expressions and friendly poses. And then put that space somewhere out in a place that's both secure and comforting and allows people to be alone. They can be alone, which is what it's designed for, or they can be with a friend or they can be with a therapist or whatever. And they can spend an hour or two out there.

It is a circular bench that's fourteen feet in diameter and there are six big animals that either sit, lie, or drape themselves over this bench. There's a giraffe, a gray wolf, a rhinoceros, a donkey, a dolphin in a tub of water, and a bear. And they're sitting and they're all posed in a way. And then it's like a big sea on the ground and then there's a space for you to pull up a chair or a wheelchair. I call it the Council of Kindness because they are kind of in a semi-circular bench or area, like a town council. And you kind of pull up your chair and then they're all looking in your direction except for one animal. A giraffe who's looking up at a hundred songbirds, wooden songbirds that are perched up in a circular ring. And it'll just be a place for people to go on a regular basis, I would imagine, just to sit and get sort of a quiet counsel or a quiet sort of, just to have company. Kind of like a kid with a teddy bear, you know? The teddy bear doesn't talk back but somehow it gives comfort to an infant, or whatever. And this would kind of be the same thing.

BK: That sounds wonderful and peaceful.[90]

---

90 For more information on Scott's projects visit www.carouselofhappiness.org and www.councilofkindness.org.

Afterword

—————

Pursuing Happiness

Years ago, when Sarah and I started dating, I was still living in Los Angeles and she was working a contract in Boulder, Colorado. We would visit back and forth, alternating between California and the Rocky Mountain State every weekend for a few months until her contract was over and my new speaking tour picked up. Each week we tried to do something special together and on one visit to Colorado, Sarah took me on a nice hike to a waterfall just outside of Boulder. I wasn't yet in as bad of shape as I was for my first time walking Mont Royal, but even then, it was difficult for me. I was low energy and easily out of breath. At the time, we chalked it up to the altitude difference, as it does sometimes take people a while to adjust to life at a mile high, but looking back I am certain it was related to my then-undiagnosed sleep apnea. I have been writing this book in Denver, and since we have been back in Colorado, I have had a strong desire to return to that same trail and see how I do on round two. Sarah and Alyssa are all dressed, snow boots and all, and waiting on me to hurry up and finish this book.

After our hike, we plan on taking Alyssa back up the mountains to Nederland for a few rounds on the Carousel of Happiness, and hopefully she can get to ride her favorite animal. Tomorrow, her uncle Jon will be coming back to town to spend Christmas with us and we have plans to take everyone to a local mall to visit Santa Claus, who I am sure Alyssa will appreciate seeing again. After we celebrate the holiday, we will be packing up our things and Sarah will no doubt be again exercising her "Car Tetris" skills as we leave Denver to hit the road for our next adventure.

I would like to end as I started, by discussing happiness. As I have shared, happiness and stress management have always been very important to me, and I sincerely hope that some of what I have shared with you here has given you some insight into how to manage stress, and the importance of taking it easy. Hopefully, some of it made you laugh in the process.

Exercise makes people happy, and for that matter so does spending time in nature. Now, I know a little girl who needs to stomp around in the snow and I can't possibly keep her waiting any longer. I just hope that we don't run into any bears, or hit traffic along the way.

Thank you for your time, and please take it easy.

Acknowledgments

There are many people who have helped me on this journey, but this book would simply not be possible if it was not for the support of my partner in life, Sarah Bollinger. In addition to being a wonderful partner and an outstanding mother, she is also an inspiration and an embodiment of nearly everything I talk about. Thank you, Sarah, for all that you do.

I would also like to thank our daughter, Alyssa, now approaching her second birthday, for not only bringing so much joy to our lives but also inspiring me to complete this book for her.

I would like to thank my brother, Jon King, for allowing me to include his story in this book and my parents, Clyde and Debbie, for their contribution to our lives and the story we are living.

I would like to thank Cuban Balestena and Scott Harrison for granting me interviews, as well as comedians Laura Hayden and Conor Kellicutt for allowing me to tell their stories.

I would like to thank my friends, psychologists Gabriel De La Rosa and Jason Schroeder, and financial advisor Jason

Goodall, for reviewing sections relating to their respective areas of expertise.

I would also like to thank everyone in my life who has taken an interest in my work and helped encourage me to pursue it, whether they are friends whom we see on a regular basis or just through our interactions on social media. In particular, I would like to acknowledge the following people for their valuable support for my work: Debbie Anderson, Liz Baker, Robin Calhoun, Daniel Dixon, Tamara Howard, John Hurst, Bill Keeshen, Kristin Kemp, Rob Lowe, Dana Masuda, Robert Mott Jr., Jim Musick, Elissa Newman, Jane Norberg, Frank Shingle, Anita and Bella Springer, Jeanne Tickle, and Misha Trubs.